YOGA
FOR COUPLES

Fun and Engaging
Exercises to Increase Flexibility and
Create a Spiritual Connection

Guillermo Ferrara

Translated by Gladis Castillo

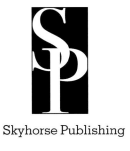

Skyhorse Publishing

Skyhorse Publishing books may be purchased in bulk at special discounts for sales promotion, corporate gifts, fund-raising, or educational purposes. Special editions can also be created to specifications. For details, contact the Special Sales Department, Skyhorse Publishing, 307 West 36th Street, 11th Floor, New York, NY 10018 or info@skyhorsepublishing.com.

Skyhorse® and Skyhorse Publishing® are registered trademarks of Skyhorse Publishing, Inc.®, a Delaware corporation.

Visit our website at www.skyhorsepublishing.com.

10 9 8 7 6 5 4 3 2 1

Library of Congress Cataloging-in-Publication Data is available on file.

Cover design by Qualcom Designs
Cover photo credit courtesy of Océano Ambar

ISBN: 978-1-63450-346-4
Ebook ISBN 978-1-63450-905-3
Printed in China

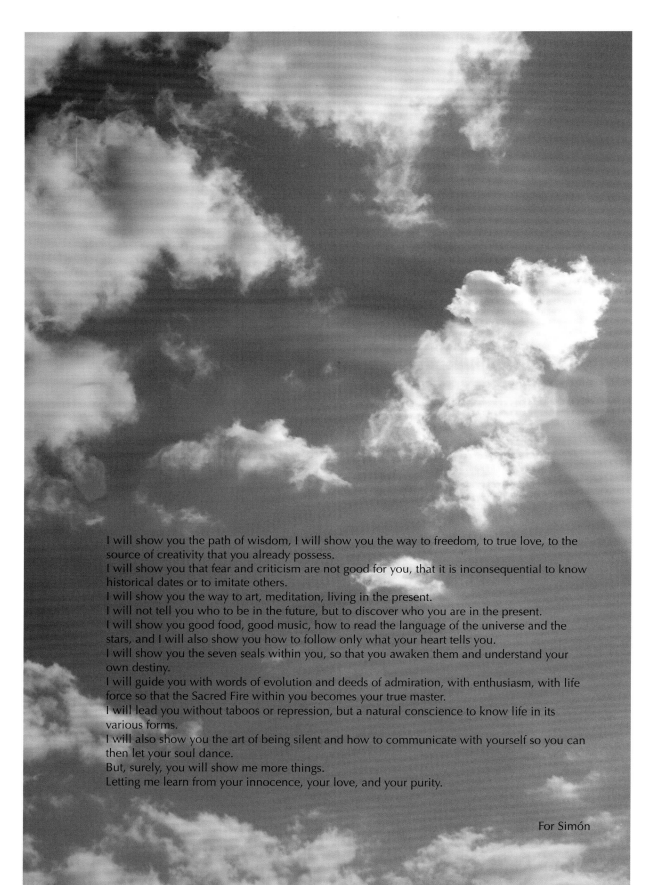

I will show you the path of wisdom, I will show you the way to freedom, to true love, to the source of creativity that you already possess.

I will show you that fear and criticism are not good for you, that it is inconsequential to know historical dates or to imitate others.

I will show you the way to art, meditation, living in the present.

I will not tell you who to be in the future, but to discover who you are in the present.

I will show you good food, good music, how to read the language of the universe and the stars, and I will also show you how to follow only what your heart tells you.

I will show you the seven seals within you, so that you awaken them and understand your own destiny.

I will guide you with words of evolution and deeds of admiration, with enthusiasm, with life force so that the Sacred Fire within you becomes your true master.

I will lead you without taboos or repression, but a natural conscience to know life in its various forms.

I will also show you the art of being silent and how to communicate with yourself so you can then let your soul dance.

But, surely, you will show me more things.

Letting me learn from your innocence, your love, and your purity.

For Simón

for Eliana Alonso,
for teaching me how to be born again, to love, and to fly . . .

ACKNOWLEDGEMENTS

I deeply wish to acknowledge those who have helped me to make this work see the light of day.

First, my editor, Jaume Rosselló, for trusting me, always bringing his vision, and to the entire technical and artistic group at Océano: Montse Vilarnau, whose "golden hands" designed this text; Mónica Campos, whose literary magnifying glass polished any defects; Laura Ogué, whose dynamisms allowed this book to reach my readers; and Esther Sanz, who provided permanent solutions.

My first yogic teachers, Dr. Fernando Estévez Griego, Hermógenes, André Van Lysebeth, and Osho, who opened the door for me toward the knowledge and the science of yoga.

My students in Argentina and Spain and all those who practice yoga while pursuing their own inner growth.

Eliana Alonso, for her faith and unconditional love since that first yoga retreat with me.

Fernando and Claudia, for giving me the space to write my first draft.

Simón, my son, who invites me to do yoga together.

Mariela, for having shared my first classes. Ricardo Aure, Elsa Tear, Dr. Simón Mina, Cristina Golato, Raúl Errezarret, and Silvia Di Gialeonardo, colleagues and friends.

Juan Cristian Ortega, for trusting my work and organizing a working trip throughout Mexico.

To the bookstore called Librería Excellence in Barcelona, for allowing me to distribute my work.

Lola Feliu and Peter Hansen, excellent human beings, friends, and professionals who helped me get past the stormy clouds with love and hospitality. Arturo and Fanny, for their light and friendship. To Gosh, vippasana master yogi and the tour group. To Mariana, my lifelong friend who helped me see the sun behind the clouds.

To all participants of the conferences that I have organized and readers of my old magazine *Terapias Naturales*.

To Barry and Robin Gibb, who continue to sing despite the pain.

To all those who trust and risk with an open heart . . . Life is a matter of enthusiasm, love of adventure, and confidence in the mystical divinity in each of us.

Contents

Introduction

This book was created with the intention of addressing a virtually undiscovered therapeutic and editorial space: yoga with a partner. It is both a compendium of yogic work and a valuable tool for those seeking a form of exercise to meet the physical and emotional needs of a couple. Yoga with a partner is like a painter who creates art on a canvas, except that here we will create art using our bodies and souls, drawing poses that inspire and uplift the spirit.

It is a dynamic, young, and modern yoga for those seeking a healthier practice using their internal and external nature, and it is also an excellent way to gain flexibility, physical strength, and emotional harmony. In the routine that many couples live, this practice can act as an "energy lifeline" by opening up significant levels of creativity that can then be applied to other aspects of daily life. And it is not exclusive to romantic partners; it can be practiced by any two people with similar weight and age.

Both fitness and aerobics are workouts that are limited to a purely physical level. Yoga with a partner aims to care for the body, its energy level, as well as its emotional and mental balance, taking into account the complete functions of the individual.

It is a free flow practice that lets you follow a path of personal awareness and enjoyment, it is a real treat for muscles, organs, and skin, and it also provides a huge increase in vitality.

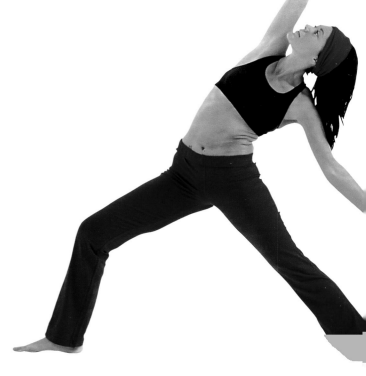

These are some basic concepts to keep in mind:
1. Willingness: to strengthen the soul
2. Discipline: to control the mind
3. Enjoyment: to rejoice the spirit

With these basic qualities you will completely transform your life and eliminate pain and disease. Use your intelligence to stay healthy, young, and live a long and prosperous life. Today many people seek conventional ideas of youth at any cost, even with surgery, ignoring the fact that there is a natural alternative through yoga (enhanced when practiced with a partner), which balances positive and negative forces into one, and benefits both genders equally. Practicing yoga with friends is recommended for young people who want to channel their energy, and for older adults who wish to explore a facet of life that involves using the innate wisdom of the body and eternal clarity of the soul.

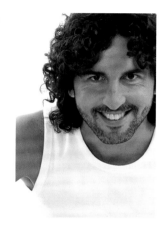

Guillermo Ferrara
Barcelona, January 2003

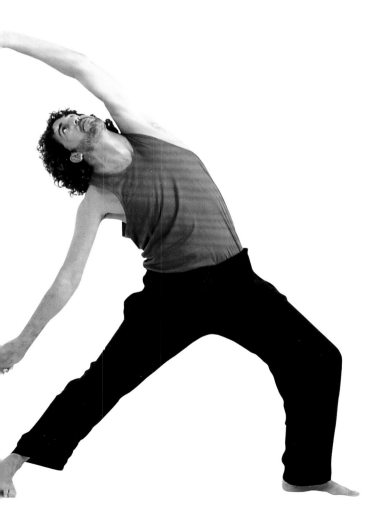

Part One

"The union of the mind to the inner sound."

is obtained by listening

Hatha Yoga Pradipika

Perceive the state of unity

It is the goal of all energy practices and paths of inner growth

Yoga with a partner merges the two polarities or life principles: the feminine and the masculine. It also works for same-sex couples, because practicing yoga brings us to a state where the sense of separation disappears.

The pace of modern life, with its hectic schedules and responsibilities, and the pressure to stay young and beautiful, cause both individuals and couples to become alienated from their inner center, feel anxiety, and live with constant stress. The energy that practicing yoga with a partner gives us tends to weaken said dividing gap and provides bioenergetic fuel in every sense: physical, emotional, mental, and spiritual.

The Universe dances eternally in the balance of its two polarities.

One of the pillars on which this practice is based is eliminating the sense of time, flowing energy between two bodies, and progressively developing flexibility. In fact, it is very interesting to note that by increasing our physical flexibility we also become increasingly flexible in our attitude and opinions.

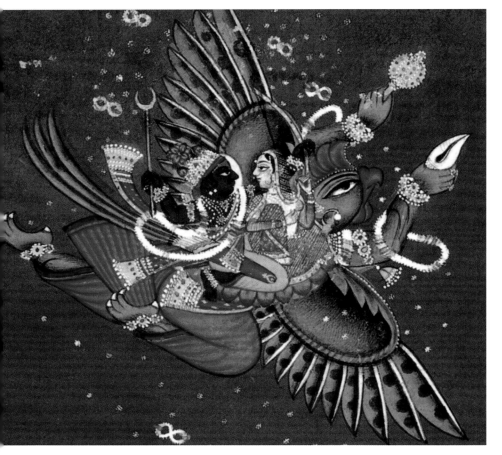

Even if two partners live a sedentary life, they should keep in mind that "A long walk begins with a single step." Both for young people, who are mentally cleaner and do not have as many bad habits, as well as for older people without a fitness routine, yoga with a partner is a tool that can be used at all levels.

There are a variety of poses and exercises, but the basic idea that must permeate every practice is to awaken a sense of unity.

The One, the Universe, or whatever you call it, is dancing forever in the balance of its two polarities. The feminine and the masculine are interrelated everywhere.

On a small scale, yoga with a partner is the representation of that magical language.

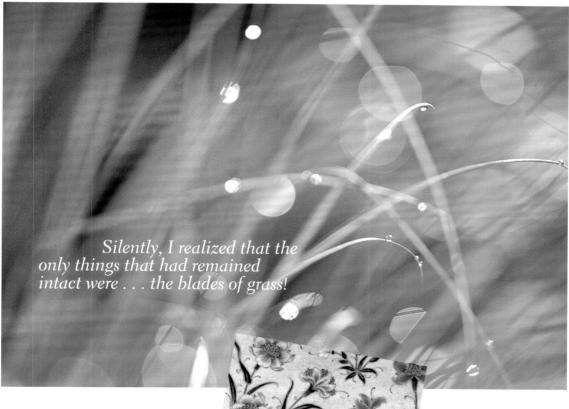

Silently, I realized that the only things that had remained intact were . . . the blades of grass!

When you practice with a partner, you are channeling and joining the sun and moon, night and day, cold and heat, winter and summer, shadow and light. If you always keep in mind the metaphysical aspect of your practice, your quality of life will improve, you will have a better relationship with your own body, with your partner, and with others, and you will begin to experience your life becoming more flexible and fluid.

It is important to learn the lessons that Mother Nature gives us: one day I saw a great storm with heavy wind and rain that knocked down trees and signs, and flooded the streets; the next day the sun came out. As I walked the streets, I saw the damage caused by the storm.

Silently, I realized that the only things that had remained intact were . . . the blades of grass! They were tiny but thanks to their flexibility, they moved back and forth and the wind could not break them; instead, large and old trees were felled despite their apparent strength. What appears to be weak has, in its nature, the quality of strength, so we should recognize that flexibility allows us to adapt to changes and that this premise intrinsically unites all things.

We must learn that what appears to be weak has, in its nature, the quality of strength.

Yoga. A divine gift
Yoga is humanity's first holistic science

Yogic vision addresses both the microcosm (man) and the macrocosm (universe). It wisely applies the laws that are within the physical body so that we may know the cosmos.

First, yoga does not study abstract problems, but it is a practical way for us to see concrete results.

The first result of practicing yoga is physical flexibility, then comes lifting energy levels, mental serenity, and emotional balance. Finally, a spiritual awakening and the desired unity with life, God, Brahma, or what we call Infinite Intelligence and Universal Love.

Etymologically, the word "yoga" comes from the Sanskrit root "yug," which translates as union and "integration." Each yogic exercise is aimed at uniting the human spirit with the divine spirit. In yoga there are no divisions, which our unconscious fails to perceive, but the spirit is always there, it is eternal.

Yoga integrates man with himself so that he can then feel complete in his existence, his personality, and his profound being. While there are various ways to practice yoga, they all have the same objective: samadhi or expansion of consciousness. This wonderful and magical event occurs when the soul vibrates in freedom and joy as it flows in harmony with the Universal Consciousness.

Whenever the practitioner performs an asana (psychophysical pose), pranayama (breathing exercise), mantra (numinous sound), or a specific meditation, he is on track towards such expansion. Yoga, as a metaphysical science, provides a manual of wisdom to men and women who feel spiritually curious without the need for religion. In fact, yoga predates religions. It is more than five thousand years old and during this period, thousands of yogis and advanced teachers have successfully practiced their yoga techniques. It is a path in which you advance through direct experience that gives you practical results.

Now in the twenty-first century, yoga is well known and practiced, its benefits are notorious, and it has spread globally. It is no longer exclusive to India and there are excellent teachers around the globe.

This book illustrates hatha and kundalini teachings using a dynamic and comprehensive approach. Yoga is no longer regarded as "gymnastics for the elderly"; it has become a conscious and intelligent discipline for every seeker.

> Yoga integrates man with himself so that he can then feel complete in his existence, his personality, and his profound being.

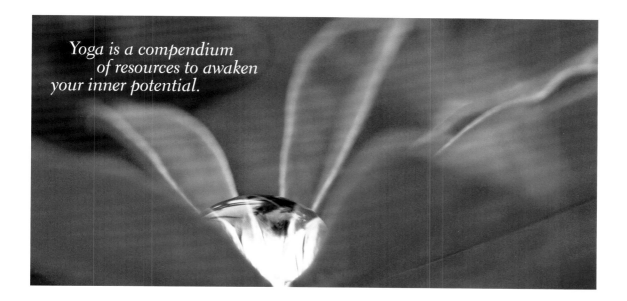

Yoga is a compendium of resources to awaken your inner potential.

"Yoga" is synonymous with "self-awareness," an ability that we develop through energetic movement. According to yoga everyone is energy in different states, from the physical body to the spiritual body. Yogic work encompasses a range of exercises and meditations that increase energy and purify the physical body, thereby opening luminous channels of the unconscious mind and inner openings where the spirit envisions a higher reality.

Yoga also integrates human beings in the world. There are misconceptions about isolation and asceticism: yoga is a resource to help you awaken your inner potential so that you have a brighter view of the world that feels integrated and unified. Yoga does not seek to separate or isolate; the days when yogis lived as hermits in the mountains are long gone. If we analyze isolation in depth, we could even think of it as a cowardly lifestyle. Contemporary yogis get involved in global issues, pay their rent, go shopping, and have children. Yogis who manage their time well can perform their daily practice (sadhana), hold a job, do housework, and meet their financial and emotional needs. Yoga is not an escape from obligations and worldly pleasures; on the contrary, these things are challenges for the soul to grow. Yoga has to be practiced all 24 hours: although the psychophysical practice and meditation take place at certain times, you can practice other forms of yoga while working, cooking, walking, breathing, or observing; it is integrated into the present moment.

Yoga has to be practiced all 24 hours.

Yoga is for anyone who feels called by their inner fire; you simply have to follow the voice of conscience, the discipline of your practice, and the cultivation of the wisdom of your soul. Yoga offers countless benefits, regardless of which branch you choose to reach samadhi.

Energy exchange
Spiritual interchange

Yoga practitioners exchange energy in a power circle (the circle is the symbol of perfection). This energy helps dissolve layers of psycho-emotional issues giving way to a spiritual openness which is simply more tolerance and patience; the opening of the fourth chakra and greater capacity to love; the increase of joy and good cheer; the feeling of the universe and the planet as living beings with continuous renewal and creation; and a deep perception of the movements of the inner world (noticing: awareness-insight).

Changes generated by opening up energy channels have effects that go beyond the physical aspect. The spirit, as a shell for the holy soul, is perfumed with positive attributes that each individual possesses; but we all have the same essence, and this is what is exposed through this practice.

The self-awareness that yoga with a partner awakens is twice extended by the energy generated by each person. Moreover, it is an intercommunication game in which you will be gently guided through the din of your mind to the peace of silence.

"Wonderful forces of love, renew the sacred fire to awaken my conscience."

Metaphysical prayer

Just as the noise of a city full of traffic, car horns, and movement is up to ninety decibels or more (resulting in an increase in the amount of blood pumped by the heart and the loss of 25 to 30 percent in your hearing ability), in a quiet place such as a field or a river, the noise level is only ten decibels.

For yogis, internal "mental noise" disappears progressively by practicing asanas, breathing techniques, bodily contact, conscious relationship with Mother Nature, and the right dynamic energy circulating prana through the meridians ("nadis").

By practicing with a partner, the chakras in one body unite with those in the other body, which greatly enhances the exchange of vitality and synchronicity.

Many people who practice yoga on a regular basis are able to develop extrasensory powers such as telepathy, knowing what their partner will say or speak at the same time, perception, intuition, and clairvoyance, which signify an opening of the upper chakras.

Bioenergetic currents that flow while performing asanas contribute to better physical, loving, and existential communication between lovers, so their practice should not be underestimated.

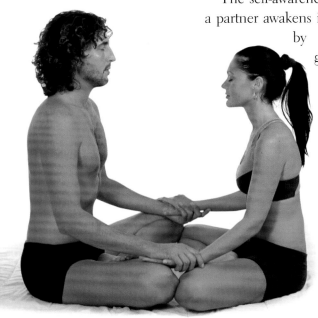

Yoga Vidya. Yoga tree

Each person can access the state of samadhi in different ways.

Vidya yoga, or "tree yoga," has many branches that rise into the sky. Thus, each individual may feel more comfortable climbing a particular path. These are the best known:

• Hatha yoga.

It is the psychophysical yoga par excellence. It is perhaps the best known in the West and it is described in this book. It is based on asanas, pranayamas, purification exercises, relaxation, and meditation.

• Kundalini yoga.

It involves doing asanas for a longer amount of time, using mantras, visualizations, mandalas, yantras (geometric diagrams for meditating), and mudras (hand gestures). It aims to stimulate psychosexual energy (called "kundalini shakti") located at the base of the spine, in the first chakra.

• Nada Yoga.

It uses only sounds or mantras, so that we access deeper levels of consciousness through vibration.

• Karma yoga.

It is yoga of action. Anything becomes yoga. It is selfless service, doing anything with the awareness that the divine is the one who acts through the doer. It is done without leaving a track.

• Raja yoga.

It is based on practicing meditation to soothe and deepen mental

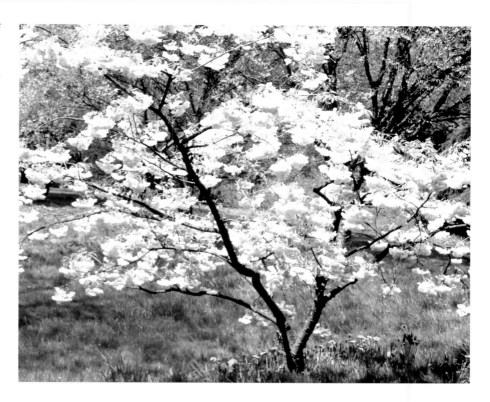

states. The creator of this system was the sage Patanjali.

• Integral Yoga.

It is a modern approach created by Sri Aurobindo that unites the basis for hatha yoga and updates them for our modern needs.

• Dhyana yoga.

Yoga of contemplation, stillness, and observation.

• Tantra yoga.

Yoga of liberation through meditative sex, mantras, internal power, pleasure (bhoga), and stimulation of the senses. It is the quintessential couple's yoga, the path of man transformed into Shiva (masculine principle) and woman

into Shakti (feminine principle). This book explores some tantric themes, but I will not dwell much on it.

• Jnana yoga.

It uses no asanas or breathing exercises. It is yoga of knowledge.

• Bhakti yoga.

Devotional yoga. Mantras are recited, rituals and meals are offered to personal divinity. Bhakti yoga also uses devotions and festive songs.

These are the paths of yoga that are most known and applied in the West. Whichever path you chose, its ultimate goal is consciously connecting the individual spirit with the Whole.

Hatha and kundalini yoga
Injections of natural energy

The Goraksashatakam says: "Everyone must resort to yoga, which is like the fruit of the Wish-Fulfilling Tree. Yogis eliminate disease by practicing poses; karmas, by controlling breathing; and mental disturbances, by withdrawing from sensations of the external world. A yogi in the highest state of samadhi is not affected by time or any other action."

"There is no greater captivity than illusion, greater strength than discipline, greater friend than wisdom, or enemy more terrible than selfishness."

Gheranda Samhita

The science of yoga is the oldest in the world. Some branches of yoga began to take shape about ten thousand years ago. Manuscripts have been found in Tibet, China, and India. Hindus have spread this discipline worldwide; from Shiva (Lord of yogis) through Patanjali (compiled classical yoga), Saraha (experimented with Tantra), Sri Aurobindo (founder of Integral

Yoga), Swami Muktananda (taught Siddha yoga), or more recently Paramahansa Yogananda, Osho, Yogi Bhajan, and thousands of guides whose teachings have spanned generations providing answers not only for the physical body, but also for spiritual fulfillment.

At first, there were only 84 yoga poses with names of animals; then came their variants that resulted in 840, and finally, with vinyasa (all possible variants of a pose) there were 84,000 asanas.

Hatha yoga is the science of balancing solar (right) and lunar (left) energy, and this state of elasticity begins by regulating the nostrils through pranayama.

Kundalini yoga is yogic energy that awakens the divinity that dwells in our body through special techniques, making it move from the source of kundalini (the sacrum) to the top of the head (the spiritual door). Those spaces that are void of any thinking, through yoga and meditation, are called "Vilamba" and when they occur, that is when kundalini rises the most.

Both types of yoga are paths towards the same goal but with different techniques and rhythms. Actually, every yoga practice seeks union and integration (Sanskrit "yug") with divine energy. Yoga is not a belief, but a practice; it is not simply read about in books, it is experienced.

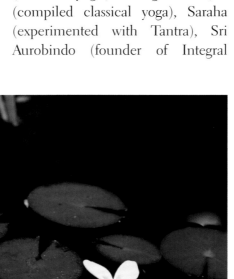

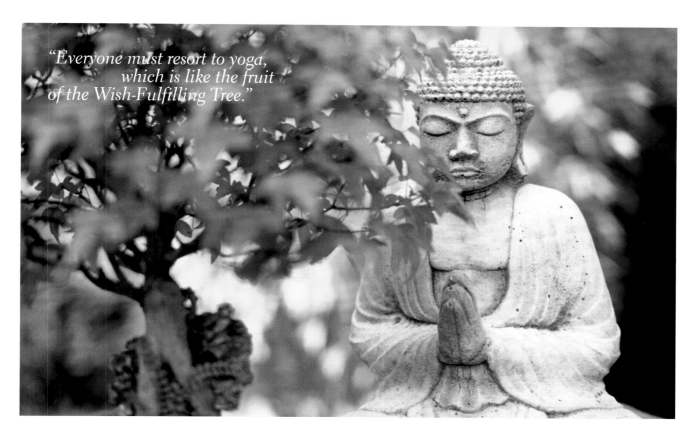

"Everyone must resort to yoga, which is like the fruit of the Wish-Fulfilling Tree."

Tantric yogis are ordinary beings who see the world as a canvas where existence creates its art. We do not escape from the world into Himalayan caves, but we boldly learn to swim between the mundane and the spiritual because there is no difference. All is one. Tantric yoga does not preach about "maya" ("illusion") because it is concerned with the real. This mix with reality is called samadhi, full union with the ocean of consciousness and eternal love.

Samadhi can be called "samprajnata samadhi" ("union with God") or "asamprajnata samadhi" ("becoming God", which is the ultimate goal of yoga).

Tantric yogis seek to follow the path of Maha Mudra ("the great symbol"), the method for obtaining one-pointedness of mind (ekagrata), which seeks mystical intuition of the true nature of existence. It is also called the "Middle Path," since it avoids any extremes. This path is not only mystics; if you are an ordinary, fashionable, or alternative person you can also enter the world of yoga. In fact, these past several years yoga has become a "trend" throughout the world.

Yoga is a complete and profound science with all kinds of benefits, but yogis can make the mistake of feeling "superior" and manifest their ego by feeling different from others, or believing that they are "the best yoga teacher"; and to prevent this from happening, we have to remember what the ancients taught us:

Yoga is a compendium of resources to awaken the potential.

Tips for Yoga

Practicing yoga will connect you with the vibration of life, it will give you fulfillment and contentment, peace, flexibility, mental relaxation, and spiritual openness. In addition to the asanas, pranayamas, mantras, mudras, and meditations, yoga is a practice that actually lasts 24 hours, so it is important to stay healthy and feel like a completely happy person.

- Keep your equanimity.
- Listen to your constant breathing; So Ham declares: "I am."
- Appreciate nature.
- Discern (viveka) what makes you grow from what does not.
- Repeat OM as medicine.
- Keep in mind that you are the master of your body and your mind.
- Elevate your brightness.

- Stay happy (you cannot have a solemn face while practicing yoga).
- Act consciously because God is protecting you at all times.
- Turn your yoga practice into a sacred hour.
- Follow your inspiration, intuition, imagination, and intelligence.

"If the eye is not blocked, there is vision. If the mind is not blocked, there is wisdom. If the spirit is not blocked, there is love."

By following the path of shastra, the path of self-control established by the sages, we get Sat ("being"), Chit ("awareness"), and Ananda ("happiness and joy"), and everything we need to live in this world. Furthermore, on a metaphysical level, yoga removes vrittis (disordered thoughts) by providing balance and eliminating karma (action of the mind), since these thoughts are transformed into ideas, ideas into beliefs, and beliefs form the samskaras, which are imprints in the subconscious that bind the cycle of birth and death.

To win the evolutionary game (lilah) our aim consists of getting rid of samsara (cycle of reincarnation) and returning to the Cosmic Home through the state of expanded consciousness, samadhi.

Yoga says that there are seven impediments, or klishas, that generate pain in the mind:

1. Addiction
2. Evil
3. Laziness and doubt
4. Apathy
5. Restlessness and anxiety
6. Fear
7. Greed, hatred, and jealousy

But there are also seven factors of enlightenment:

1. Attention
2. Inquiry of reality
3. Energy
4. Joy
5. Quiet
6. Concentration
7. Fairness

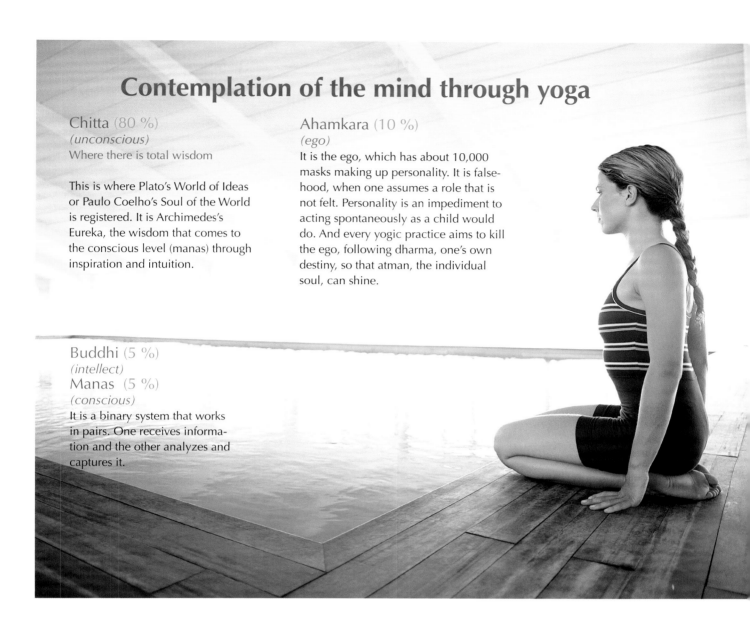

Contemplation of the mind through yoga

Chitta (80 %)
(unconscious)
Where there is total wisdom

This is where Plato's World of Ideas or Paulo Coelho's Soul of the World is registered. It is Archimedes's Eureka, the wisdom that comes to the conscious level (manas) through inspiration and intuition.

Ahamkara (10 %)
(ego)
It is the ego, which has about 10,000 masks making up personality. It is falsehood, when one assumes a role that is not felt. Personality is an impediment to acting spontaneously as a child would do. And every yogic practice aims to kill the ego, following dharma, one's own destiny, so that atman, the individual soul, can shine.

Buddhi (5 %)
(intellect)
Manas (5 %)
(conscious)
It is a binary system that works in pairs. One receives information and the other analyzes and captures it.

Yoga is a journey toward self-knowledge. As noted by Jiddu Krishnamurti—whom I admire for believing more in the individual than in organizations, which are ultimately a group of individuals:

"If you want to discover the truth in that vital process which is your own life, not just the superficial part, but the entire process of your being, then it is relatively easy.

"If you really wish to know yourself, you will have to inquire deeply, give your heart and mind to it. Then, without condemnation or justification, you can have independent thoughts and feelings; and following every thought and every feeling as it arises, you find a peace that does not come from willingness or discipline, but it is the result of having no problems, no contradiction. It is like a lake that becomes calm and serene at nightfall when there is no longer any wind; and when the mind is calm, that which is immeasurable manifests itself."

Secrets of energy

"Energy is every phenomenon that produces movement"

Just as a car uses energy from fuel but still needs a driver to steer it, energy within the multiple bodies in each individual needs to be steered consciously in order to get the best results.

When kundalini energy is released, it is important to know what to do with it. We have to have a creative outlet for it to flow, where it can manifest without any blockages.

The first step is purification, which can be done by changing our eating habits (intelligently giving our body what it needs) and practicing with all yogic tools: special breathing, active and passive meditations, and conscious visualization of the chakras. You can also sing a mantra, which are numinous sounds that resonate spiritually.

After purification, kundalini energy will open up through the central duct and rise up. Please note that this process is not fast; it requires years of training. Each individual, according to his or her own development, will require practice for a certain amount of time. There are no specific or general formulas to predict when kundalini will rise completely; it is a conscious and individual process, although there are very powerful group exercises to help energy rise.

Planetary kundalini Shakti is awakening in this era where more and more people feel the need to practice meditation, yoga, and other methods to achieve inner growth. Kundalini is the divine spark inside the human body and as it moves from the first to the seventh chakra, it mixes with spiritual energy that gives life to everything, thus producing cell regeneration (which are filled with energy and light) as well as spiritual regeneration (that feeds on conscience, joy, and expansion).

Energy is the divine spark inside the human body and as it moves from the first to the seventh chakra, it mixes with spiritual energy that gives life to everything, thus producing cell regeneration (which are filled with energy and light) as well as spiritual regeneration (that feeds on conscience, joy, and expansion).

A person may feel changes due to moving energy:

- Releasing several layers of energy may make it move up from the sacrum to the top of the head, resulting in a magnificent state of energizing spiritual bliss and peace.

- Increased physical strength, new metaphysical interpretations, unlimited creativity, and enlightened states of consciousness.

- People with blockages may experience pain due to not being completely purified. All pain is blocked energy, so it is important to undergo a cleansing process to prevent energy from getting stuck at any point.

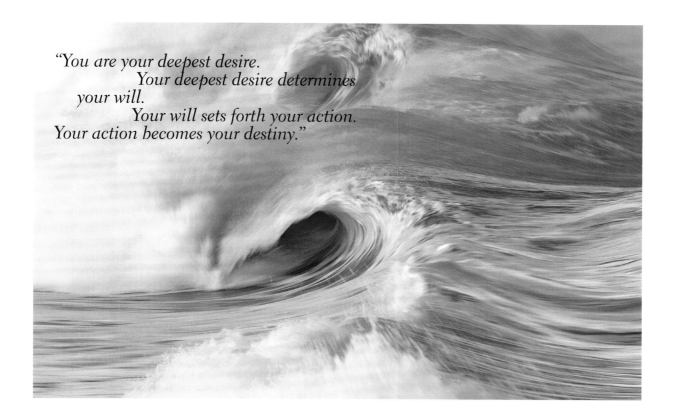

*"You are your deepest desire.
Your deepest desire determines
your will.
Your will sets forth your action.
Your action becomes your destiny."*

Someone who continuously works with energy is more likely to lead and channel their energy, feed off it, and enjoy its stimulating effect on vital energy flow and emotional functions.

Internal powers of the 7 chakras

Practicing yoga with a partner expands the senses and awakens the inner powers of the chakras.

The seven chakras are energy wheels that make up human consciousness. These circular transmitters connect the physical world of the individual with the world of energy. Each chakra exists at an astral level, but they correspond with glands of the endocrine system. Chakras are stimulated through yoga practice that makes them function better and which eventually helps us obtain siddhis.

Siddhis or extrasensory powers that exist in each chakra are not an end goal; rather, they come from practicing while aiming to reach samadhi stage.

Chakras do not always work properly because they can be closed, blocked, or over-stimulated.

As a yogic aphorism says, "The same key that locks the door can also open it"—but on the other side.

Activating the chakras is the foundation for practicing yoga with a partner and many variations of yoga.

Practicing yoga daily increases chakra energy.

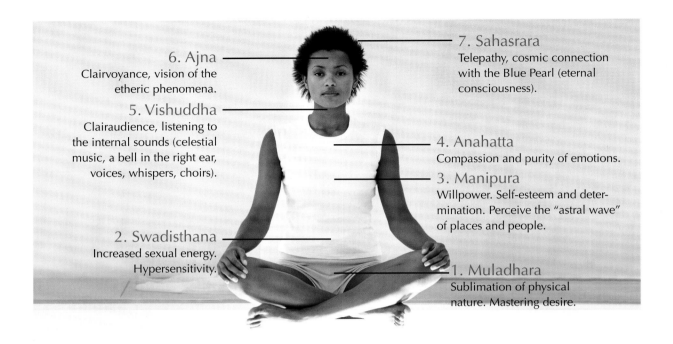

6. Ajna
Clairvoyance, vision of the etheric phenomena.

5. Vishuddha
Clairaudience, listening to the internal sounds (celestial music, a bell in the right ear, voices, whispers, choirs).

2. Swadisthana
Increased sexual energy. Hypersensitivity.

7. Sahasrara
Telepathy, cosmic connection with the Blue Pearl (eternal consciousness).

4. Anahatta
Compassion and purity of emotions.

3. Manipura
Willpower. Self-esteem and determination. Perceive the "astral wave" of places and people.

1. Muladhara
Sublimation of physical nature. Mastering desire.

The diagram represents the powers that each person holds inside.

Yoga helps us attain siddhis by practicing meditation, asanas, sex without ejaculation, pranayama, mantras, stimulating kundalini and chakras, fasting, and having contact with fire.

A Siddha Yogi is one who has obtained paranormal abilities and has ascended above physical limitations. Readers may doubt these paranormal attainments, but they may experience it for themselves through dedication and by opening and using internal channels. We have an intelligent awareness and several cell sub-consciences that can be used to open gates or siddhis, depending on the person. No one who seeks to attain siddhis for power and to satisfy their ego while ignoring samadhi will get them. Ego cannot access paranormal powers; it is the soul's natural ability.

The range of powers attained depends on awakening the chakras.

The implosion of kundalini into the sahasrara implies very intense and rich experiences that each individual experiences in their own way. Experiencing it is beyond words, and that is why tantric yoga can help us explore it.

This awakening occurs because yoga practice leads to the knowledge of energy, which is a science that has been in practice for thousands of years and that now we have the chance to experience for ourselves.

Practicing yoga with a partner feeds the soul, reveals the constraints of conscience to see with the mind's eye, and produces the greatest transformation in humans, the spiritual rebirth altogether.

And how are chakras activated? Besides practicing asanas, mantras, and meditation, you must apply pranayama techniques through breathing.

And we must activate our chakras because they have lost their ancestral power; in the past, the human body was created with cells capable of absorbing and consuming ninety percent of light and cosmic forces received. Later, cells began to deteriorate until they could only absorb and consume five to ten percent of energy, and this was when it began to lose sexual energy.

The science of pranayama says that breathing is actively done using one nostril then the other (switching approximately every hour and 48 minutes); we only breathe for ten minutes using both nostrils, and then the cycle starts again. You can check this very easily: place a finger over one nostril and exhale loudly, then do the other: you will notice that more air comes out of one than the other.

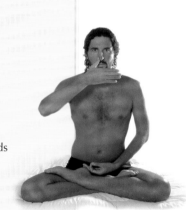

Activities that are benefited

Right nostril. Solar
- Initiate actions and physical effort
- Enjoy erotic passion
- Seduction of women
- Share hugs
- Have sex
- Play sports
- Sell something
- Bathe
- Eat

Left nostril. Lunar
- Artistic activities
- Study and paint
- Plant or sow
- Make a living
- Buy something
- Prepare food
- Travel and visit friends
- Enter a house

Many Yogic teachers have described such experiences, just as Swami Muktananda does here:

"By raising kundalini to the sahasrara we begin to experience a divine effulgence. There are a thousand knots in the sahasrara, which glow with the radiance of a thousand suns but rather than burn, its light is cool. This light is so powerful that when it is revealed to you, you have no strength to endure it. When I saw that brilliance within myself, I collapsed because I could not withstand its intensity. In the center of that effulgence, there is a fascinatingly beautiful and tiny light—a blue pearl—and when your meditation deepens, you start to see it shining and beaming. Sometimes it comes out through your eyes and stays in front of you. It moves at the speed of light and it is so subtle that as it passes through the eye, the eye does not feel it.

"The vision of the Blue Pearl is the most significant of all the experiences I have described. Everyone should see this blue pearl at least once. The scriptures describe the Blue Pearl as the divine light of consciousness that dwells within each of us. It is the real way of being. Our most intimate reality, God living within us. The Blue Pearl is subtler than the subtle. It is as big as a sesame seed. And despite being so small it is very big, because it contains this world of animate and inanimate things. The banana tree seed is so small that if you take it between your fingers and crush it, it disappears. However, if you plant the seed, it sprouts a huge tree with endless banana seeds. Likewise, within the Blue Pearl there are millions and millions of universes. It contains the entire cosmos."

Yoga meditations
for personal growth

For modern humans it is almost impossible to enter the field of meditation, inner silence, without first knowing what causes problems, fear, trauma, and conflict. We need to know where the voices of ego are so we can cross into silence, where only the soul and the one exist.

Meditation calms the mind and declutters our thoughts through a state of inner balance that leads to purification.

Practicing yoga is essential because it is impossible to obtain results without it. First there will be a few minutes of inner emptiness and clarity, but these will increase until you can meditate at any moment and you will always feel centered.

Meditation will push out of your life anything that does not help you grow: bad habits, weaknesses, insecurity, laziness . . . The more you practice meditation, the closer you are to your true being, your will, your consciousness awakening, and love as high energy. Freedom is within each of us, but so is slavery . . . You decide. Are you a prisoner of your schedule? Do you dislike your job? Do your relationships not work out as you would have hoped? Everything is limited to the boundaries of the ego. Beliefs like "I cannot afford to change jobs" or "I hope to find someone to love me" generate a mental rigidity without liberty or happiness.

The more you meditate, the closer you get to truth and happiness within your soul. And you get more power, certainty, enthusiasm, and energy.

Meditation will change you and make you grow, and change the vibration of your surroundings, your life, and your experiences. You will attract what you send out, so if you give out peace and joy, life will give you back this enhanced vibration twofold.

The ultimate goal of meditation is samadhi, enlightenment of consciousness, personal evolution for those who realize that they are fish swimming in divine waters. It is the "eureka" that raises awareness.

There are different degrees of enlightenment, from a bright idea to the final samadhi of oneness with the whole. As Osho says: "When you become enlightened, all existence becomes enlightened.

Advice

- All meditations are done on an empty stomach or two hours after eating.
- Before meditating, do some relaxation in the early morning or after practicing yoga with your partner.
- If you can, do the meditations wearing little or no clothes.
- Do not fight your own body: meditate in a comfortable position.
- Do not fight your own mind: let thoughts pass by like clouds moved by the wind.

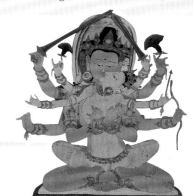

If you are in the dark, then all existence is in the dark. It all depends on you."

There are a thousand fallacies about meditation when in reality it is very simple: meditation is awareness. It is not about reciting a mantra or using a rosary; these are just simple hypnotic methods that can provide some relaxation, but they can never reveal truth to us.

Meditation means transforming innocence into consciousness. Only a tenth of our brain is conscious, and nine-tenths are unconscious; therefore, only a small part of our mind, a thin layer, has light, and the rest is dark. The challenge is to grow that little light until the entire "home" is flooded with light, and there are no corners left in the dark.

Shared breathing meditation

This meditation is also called circle of light.

Sit comfortably in Yab-Yum position (man sitting cross-legged and woman on top of him with her legs spread) and join in an embrace. Begin to breathe through the nose softly, deeply, loudly, and with the same rhythm.

This meditation allows physical boundaries to disappear and you feel as though you are a circle of light through breathing. For at least 45 minutes breathe without stress, thoughts, or desires. Little by little your breathing will become one and you will both merge with the Whole, experiencing spiritual unity.

Thus, everything becomes extraordinary, the mundane becomes sacred, and the little things in life begin to have an importance that we could have never imagined. Stones begin to seem as beautiful as diamonds and all of our existence becomes illuminated.

Opening the heart

Lying on a blanket, meditate for seven cycles and then your partner will do the same. The goal is to open the fourth chakra, the center of loving energy.

For several minutes, inhale deeply and then exhale to expel all the air from the lungs. When you feel you no longer have air, hold it without breathing as long as you can. Gradually the lungs gain flexibility and expand their capacity. Breathe normally whenever you feel the need for air and you will feel how energy flows directly to the chest chakra; your heart will open and blossom. Repeat this process seven times.

Like all meditations, it is better to do it on an empty stomach. You can do it four or five times a day. You will feel a source of loving energy that constantly flows in the chest area, and your individual heart will be able to connect with the universal heart, making your life more passionate, free, and loving.

Meditation of the third eye or soul

Sit comfortably in meditation pose or in a chair with your feet flat on the floor; close your eyes, and massage your third eye and then your partner's. Make a clockwise motion (viewed from the front) and then very gently make an upward pressing motion with one hand. Energy between the eyes will awaken and flow. You will immediately feel a sense of openness, but if you do not then continue making this motion as you gaze toward the sky activating this area. Visualize a point between the eyebrows, keep your eyes closed, and channel all your energy to that spot. You will awaken and channel sexual energy and intuition.

Do this meditation for an hour, without abrupt interruption, and finish slowly. You can accompany this meditation with the sound of a gong or a Tibetan bowl.

At this point, your soul leaves the body and travels to other dimensions, providing a clear view of reality. This meditation increases self-awareness because it reveals your true nature and provides instant existential knowledge that is not intellectual.

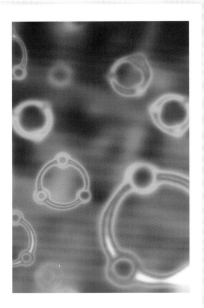

Full moon meditation

The Moon rules and influences the feminine qualities of nature. It powers intuition, inspiration, perception, and everything related to the creative process as long as you are responsive and harmonized; otherwise, it increases violence and uncontrolled passions.

The moon is linked to the water element, so it affects the emotional and sensory system. During a full moon, our energy is very strong and powerful, so we need to be in a harmonious state in order to receive its benefit on the body, mind, and emotions.

When the Moon is crescent, observe it every night for at least thirty minutes.

During a full moon, drink at least three liters of mineral water during the day, and on an empty stomach take a shower to remove any negative energy. Then sit facing the moon in meditation pose, and begin to breathe deeply, keeping your eyes closed, for at least ten minutes. When you have silenced your mind, open your eyes and watch the moon as if you were seeing it for the first time. Concentrate on its circular shape and receive energy from the sun through it; feel its light and clarity. Be receptive and perceive how it illuminates the entire sky with its mantle. Let its energy flow through you, with the rhythm of the night. When at least thirty minutes have gone by, close your eyes and look at it from inside using your third eye.

This meditation increases creativity, intuition, sensuality, and sexuality channeled throughout the body, and brings you closer to the magical side of nature.

Use the power of the moon to stimulate energy and consciousness. You can enhance your ability to fulfill a desire or complete a project if you do this meditation for seven consecutive days. Do not forget to breathe deeply to receive lunar energy through inhalation.

Sun meditation

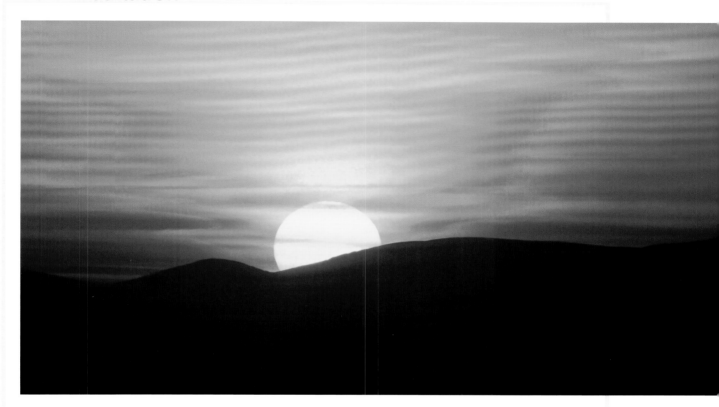

The Sun allows life to exist on Earth; so, why shouldn't we be grateful to it? The Sun is five and a half times as big as the distance from the Earth to the Moon; can you imagine something so immense? Tanning is a simple consequence of exposure to sunlight; so do not pay attention to this insignificant fact but rather try to use the Sun's energy creatively. The Sun also emits prana, vital energy that enters our body through breathing. The Sun is a magical tool because prana responds to the mind; that is, the sun can help us use that energy to generate power and fulfill wishes. It is best to meditate on the beach or out on a field, naked, and lying on the sand or grass (cover your head with a hat or cloth), but you can do it sitting down with your spine upright and facing north to absorb energy or to the east to show devotion. Concentrate on the sun as though you were two Egyptian pharaohs worshiping the Sun. Relax and let its fire consume your thoughts.

Feel the heat in your skin and how energy enters through three breaths:

1. Abdominal.
Inflate and deflate the abdominal area for fifteen minutes.

2. Complete.
Use the lower, middle, and upper torso as you breathe for thirty minutes.

3. Retention.
Take a deep breath; hold it for ten to fifteen seconds. Do this seven times and then slowly come back to normal abdominal breathing.

You must fully concentrate on the Sun's energy; how it nourishes your cells, chakras, energy, and nervous system. If either of you has heart problems, you should not hold your breath; only do steps 1 and 3. Do not go past the recommended amount of time. The best time to practice it is early in the morning (sattva guna), which is best for purification.

Conditions for practice
"Make yoga a sacred and pleasant rite"

Many people complain that they lack time when in fact if they divide their day into three equal parts they can get eight hours for sleep, eight for work and . . . eight hours free! However, if you really have little free time, you can practice yoga with your partner for half an hour in the morning and half an hour at the end of the day.

Some people look at pictures of yoga poses in my previous books and exclaim: "Ah! I used to be able to get into this pose two years ago . . ." They should know that no asana is cumulative; that is, it is only when you practice it that it helps your body and mind.

Everything is customizable to each couple and laziness is the worst enemy, so the most important thing is the idea that if something is beneficial for us, we should continue doing it.

There are some things to keep in mind as we practice yoga with a partner:

"Think of your yoga practice as a sacred encounter, not an obligation."

Flexibility

"Be like a blade of grass, or a river bed coming down from the mountain, which adapt themselves to the evolution of the forces of nature."

Not all bodies are equal in terms of elasticity and flexibility. You must respect your limitations and your partner's limitations because otherwise you could experience pain and injury.

Flexibility is something that is gradually acquired. Just as a seed takes time to germinate and become a great tree, a neophyte who is just beginning to practice must have patience ("science of peace") so that his muscles, bones, and joints can take shape through exercise.

If you look at a child—or remember back to when you were a child—you will notice that children possess a high degree of natural flexibility. And no wonder, since their "vehicle" mileage is 0. We lose this condition as we grow older through lack of exercise, poor posture, rigid personality, sedentary lifestyle, etc. Being flexible has many benefits at many levels. A sedentary lifestyle and bad habits are detrimental to both our body and mind. If you want to have a long life and a vigorous old age, practice flexibility daily.

Care for your body with pleasure so that you can stay healthy.

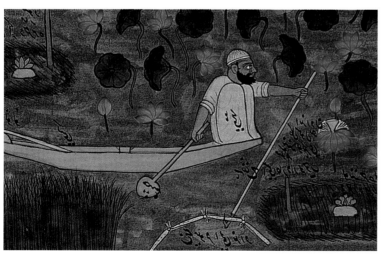

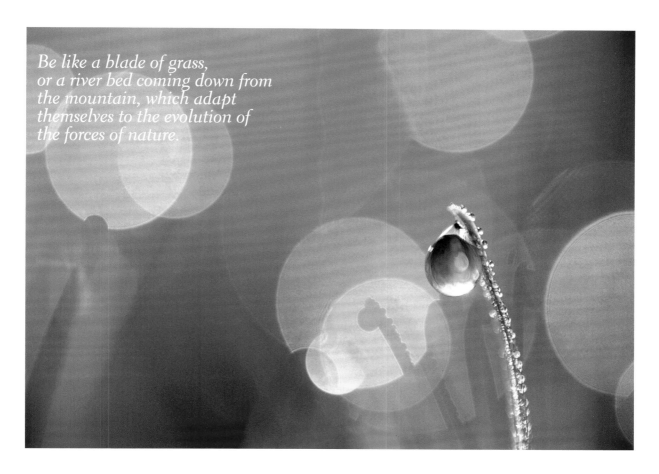

Be like a blade of grass, or a river bed coming down from the mountain, which adapt themselves to the evolution of the forces of nature.

Age, weight, and height

"Yoga will make you stop aging through cellular stimulation and recharge, which will give your face a healthy and bright appearance, regulate your weight, and give you your best possible posture."

To practice yoga with a partner, it is important that both persons have similar body weight and height.

Since many asanas require that the backbone be subjected to specific movements and exercise, and we use our hands and arms for support during asanas, there should not be more than a foot (35 cm) difference in height between the partners. In terms of weight, the difference should not exceed 77 pounds (35 kilograms).

Age is not a major requirement if the older partner is more advanced in yoga, remains in good shape, or practices sports.

You can also take care of your body by practicing with your partner or a friend who has a similar build to yours and let yourself be surprised by the wonders of yoga.

To practice yoga with a partner, it is important that both persons have similar body weight and height.

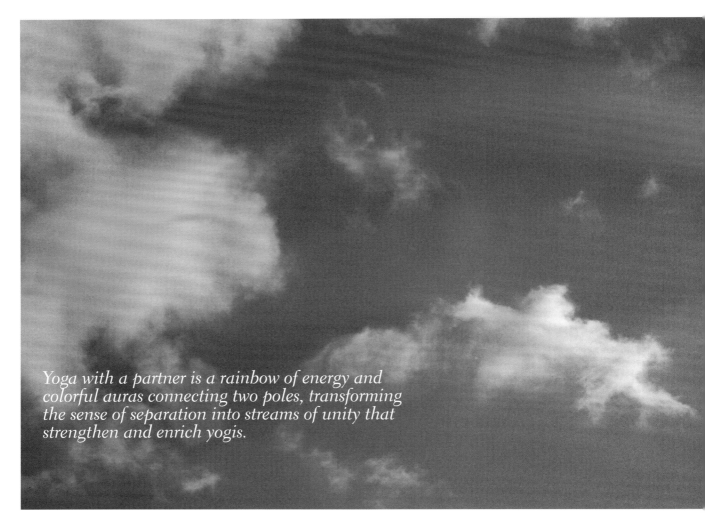

Yoga with a partner is a rainbow of energy and colorful auras connecting two poles, transforming the sense of separation into streams of unity that strengthen and enrich yogis.

Permanence and mobility

"All changes in nature are mild and require time; only disasters are sudden."

You will come across poses that need to be held for several minutes, while others only take a few seconds; it is important that you recognize their stimulus on a particular body part as you do them.

There are dynamic and still asanas; they both have an effect on your body and on your chakras, stimulating and interrelating energy from one practitioner to another.

Do your dynamic asanas in the morning to "awaken" your body and mind; on the other hand, twilight is best for increasing the duration of each asana, giving greater flexibility to the spine and joints.

Interaction

"Practicing yoga with a partner will reinforce your bond."

When energies are moving, there can be two basic principles: attraction or repulsion. A person can either lure or repel you.

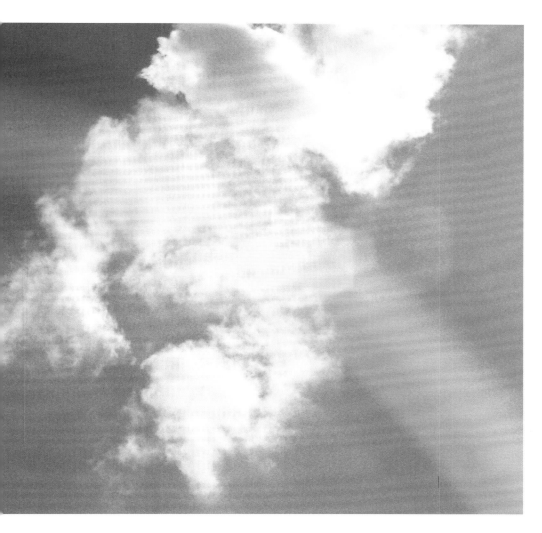

Yogis do not
need to be
a romantic
couple; they
can marvel at
the waves of
universal love.

The energy flow that emanates allows them to merge and fuse, producing a yogic power circuit.

Both the fusion of magnetism (male) and electricity (female) bring forth a stream of energy (life).

And this life can generate an interaction that over time will become a bond, which comes from sharing energy connectivity through balancing and speaking with the chakras.

If you practice with someone who is not your partner, be forewarned: high energy is no other than . . . love!

Two practitioners can easily come to love one another through the energy bridge they create. Yoga with a partner is a rainbow of energy and colorful auras connecting two poles, transforming the sense of separation into streams of unity that strengthen and enrich yogis.

However, since there are three kinds of love: filial (among family and friends), eros (between lovers), and agape (universal), yogis do not need to be a romantic couple; they can marvel at the waves of universal love (which includes absolutely everything) or shared friendship.

Benefits of yoga with your partner
Yoga gives you the secret to well-being

Simon Mundy presents a beautiful description of the benefit of practicing yoga: "When the sun is low on the horizon and it is projected onto someone who is standing, it enlarges their shadow on the surface of the earth. As the sun moves up across the sky, the shadow becomes smaller, and once the sun is in the center of the sky, the shadow vanishes completely. What is yoga, if not this elevation of man's (and woman's) internal sun until there is no shadow left in their inner world? And when this sun shines fully on our inner world and banishes all darkness, a luminous state of clarity, truth, joy, and serenity emerges."

By practicing hatha and kundalini yoga, the body becomes agile, young, supple, and healthy. In fact, yoga helps keep the body in good health well into old age.

Advantages of practicing yoga

- Closeness between partners.
- Increased muscle flexibility that doubles when stimulated by an external force.
- Chakras are recharged through interaction and contact.
- Increased body heat.

- Creating an interior space for intimacy.
- Internal intuitive understanding of laws governing the universe.
- Using a conscious feeling of unity to eliminate any sense of separation.

- Renewed desire to play.
- Awakening telepathy.
- Activating creativity.
- Internalization and introspection.
- Energy exchange through yin/yang currents.
- Awakening trust.
- Acquiring greater muscle strength.
- Loving connection.
- Improved breathing capacity.
- Attaining discipline and joy, not as something imposed or routine.
- Toning the body and improving facial appearance.
- Improving blood flow to the heart, brain, and nervous system.
- Detoxifying cells and eliminating fatigue.
- Opening channels of spiritual communication.

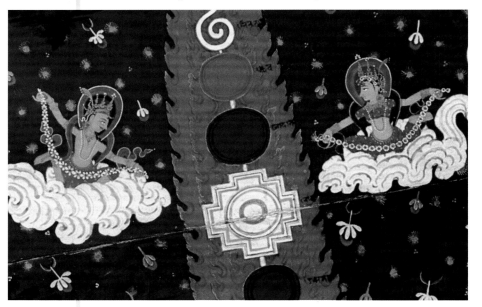

Yoga emphasizes maintaining health to prevent physical disorders and diseases, cultivating a harmonious lifestyle according to the laws of nature, and getting energy from the sun, the moon, food, air, and prana, which are particles of pure energy found in the air. (More about prana in the "Pranayama" chapter.)

The body, therefore, is the start and the field where the game of life is played. Within the body there is transcendent existential opportunity for spiritual enlightenment.

Many cultures are not set up to support the natural state of the body and this causes many people to suffer from overweight, pain, inflexibility, or diseases. Why do people overeat, and abuse alcohol and drugs? Why doesn't the world live in a state of ecstasy? I think there is a very basic awareness of how the body works and the enormous energy it stores. We tend to overemphasize individuality, but we do not focus enough on our internal energy. Not appreciating our own body is a self-destructive behavior caused by lack of self-love and low levels of affection for others, as well as poor physical posture or somatization of emotional and psychological problems, which create barriers, or what W. Reich referred to as "shells" —defensive mechanisms that generate pain and deformities.

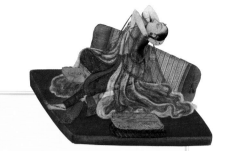

Changes observed in yoga practitioners

- They stop taking sleeping pills.
- They have more energy during the day.
- They do better at work.
- They stop feeling anxiety.
- They connect better with their own emotions and with others.
- They stay healthy and in a good mood.
- They develop the sense of observation without forming attachment.
- They fix specific problems, such as difficulty breathing.
- They become more flexible with their body and their personality.

Tantric yoga is a path toward the soul, beginning with a complete workout on the body, emphasizing vegetarian and sattvic diet, channeling vital energy to charge our chakras, and stretching through asanas so that the meridians are able to carry qi or prana.

I remember when I started practicing, more than twelve years ago, when I was done exercising alone I was in such a blissful state that I would start crying, full of emotion; I almost always did relaxing poses with tears in my eyes. Now, many of my students have experienced significant changes thanks to yoga, and I notice the many changes that yoga practitioners undergo as they continue to practice diligently.

"For he who is moderate, the discipline of yoga frees him from all evil."
BHAGHAVAD GITA

Finding time and space
8 hours for work, 8 for sleep and . . . 8 hours free!

A lot of people complain about "not having enough time" when in fact, time is a concept created by man. In ancient times, a day had more than 24 hours and for aboriginal people whose living was closely associated to natural cycles, there was neither stress nor clocks!

We created time, so we should be masters of our own time, not its slave.

Instead of watching so much television, working, or focusing on what others are doing, use that time to practice yoga and stop making excuses. And if you have children, you can have them practice right along with you as you teach them that yoga is important for their health and well-being. We choose for ourselves. We are free to decide whether we take care of ourselves or fall into a barren swamp of comfort, inactivity, inertia or, failing that, too much work.

Many people will tell me: "I used to practice yoga two years ago and it was very good," and when I ask them why they did not continue, they give me a thousand excuses. Keep in mind something that is very important: yoga is not cumulative, meaning that unless we practice it regularly, we lose any benefits the asanas can give us.

Practicing two or three times a week (seven days would be ideal) is necessary to move forward. Find a special time to share it with your partner or friend and you will see how each day feels better.

> "Set aside a time of day that is sacred for your practice; gradually that moment will begin to extend, until you feel that every moment of the day is sacred."

Laziness versus willpower

Laziness is part of the ego, but your willpower turns your soul into a king. This is a critical point in your practice and everyone has had to face this duality and fight through it. By finding your center and acting, feeling, and thinking with your soul, there is simply no room for laziness. Your willingness works to benefit your soul and it is able to recognize anything that is not beneficial, even if it means making more of an effort.

Life is a balance between relaxation and effort. Extremes of any kind are bad.

This is personal work: find your willpower and put it to use; you will communicate positively with your soul, which will guide you to the path you need most. Someone who has willpower—which is something very different from being stubborn—becomes powerful, reliable, strong, and also brave.

> "Tomorrow is an excuse for those who have no desire, and joy for the ego of laziness."

We created time, so we should be masters of our own time, not its slave.

Intimacy

One of the biggest advantages of practicing yoga with a partner is the deep level of intimacy that you will share. And intimacy is a whisper of the divine.

If you and your yoga partner are romantically involved, the intensity of your connection will increase twofold. As modern Adam and Eve you will recreate your own paradise, full of magic, complicity, and empathy, moving toward communicating without words, with the language of the soul.

Intimacy calms anxiety and brings both partners into a state where there is no time and there are no thoughts—a state of mental emptiness and conscious presence that lets you surrender into a state of deep relaxation and peace.

Intimacy eliminates egos, which are identity and individuality, and strengthens the soul with love.

The ego possesses, it does not love, and practicing yoga with a partner helps you create a path towards love, unity, intimacy, and balance by using your consciousness. The I in each person loses its boundaries and it expands to the point that knowledge, the knower, and the known become one.

By becoming intimate, both partners get to know themselves and are able to recognize everything in their hearts. The external and the internal become the same: a feeling of unity and love that is the One.

"Intimacy is like a delicate flower that needs care so it becomes more beautiful day by day."

Personal growth

- There are two types of growth: physical and spiritual. According to Mantak Chia: "Initially the human body was created with cells capable of absorbing and consuming ninety percent of light and cosmic forces received. Later, our cells began to deteriorate until they could only absorb and consume five to ten percent of energy, and we began to lose sexual energy."
- For tantra, it is known that psychosexual energy (kundalini) causes internal alchemy, transforms the psyche, promotes creativity, and deepens spirituality. This type of evolution occurs first at a physical level (with changes ranging from improved bowel movements to better mental clarity and proper organ functioning) and then develops into a spiritual transformation.
- Osho declares: "When someone reaches consciousness, enlightenment, he is completely outside of the realm of cause and effect. He becomes totally unpredictable, living every moment." And that is because yoga flows into the ocean of consciousness, of free and individual spiritual change. By sharing this journey with your partner, your growth is more powerful and enjoyable.
- Practice transforms fear into love, insecurity into high esteem, laziness into willpower, uncertainty into absolute confidence, confusion into mental clarity, and existential emptiness gives way to using the gifts of the soul.

"Our ego is terrified by what our soul craves."

ANA AVRUJ

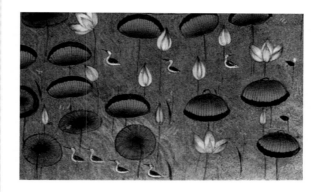

Doing wonders for the body
"The human body is a divine invention"

Take care of your body and it will react positively to the stimulus of yoga. The human body is a complex, orderly, and marvelous laboratory that seamlessly blends its systems and functions. A tantric principle states: "He who knows the reality of the body knows the reality of the universe."

Yoga comprises a range of psycho-physical and spiritual techniques to attain harmony and transcendence (samadhi). Asanas or yoga poses make energy flow through the meridians, stimulate the chakras, and relieve muscle stiffness, providing a high degree of flexibility. These poses are accompanied by breathing methods and a silent mental attitude.

The body is heard, valued, and prepared, and the temple is treated with love and care. Postures (most of which make references to animals) are held in contemplation for a positive effect.

The obvious end goal in hatha yoga is unifying polarities, preparing the body for consciousness.

Yoga empowers us as practitioners because it activates our latent sexual power that resides in the first chakra: flowing Shakti energy that moves up toward Shiva on top of the head. Between these two extremes, life flows through the spine and the seven chakras. To this end, we practice asanas, which are certain poses that tend to have precise effects on bodily functions, personality,

energy, mind, and emotional state. By mastering the body we are able to master the mind.

Every asana or yoga pose requires strict adherence to technicalities and some prerequisites such as steadfastness, permanence, comfort, and stillness. Over the centuries, thousands of yogis have personally verified the effectiveness and scope of each asana, its effects, and its benefits.

Almost all asanas are available to anyone; practicing yoga only requires enjoyable consistency without competition or goals. You do not need to be able to place your forehead on your knee in the first practice; just be aware that you are taking care of your body.

There are thousands of yoga poses (although eighty-four are the most traditional and around twenty are the most basic) and they are named after animals, plants, scholars, heroes, sages, and divinities, or according to the individual characteristics of each asana.

> "The first step of the spiritual ladder is the human body."
>
> TANTRIC PRINCIPLE

Respect for the body

The human body is an immense reservoir of secrets and powers; therefore, we first need to know it and then take care of it. Tibetan lamas claim that being reborn in a body from the astral plane is the most difficult.

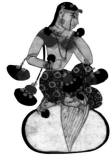

"The body is a laboratory for spiritual enlightenment."

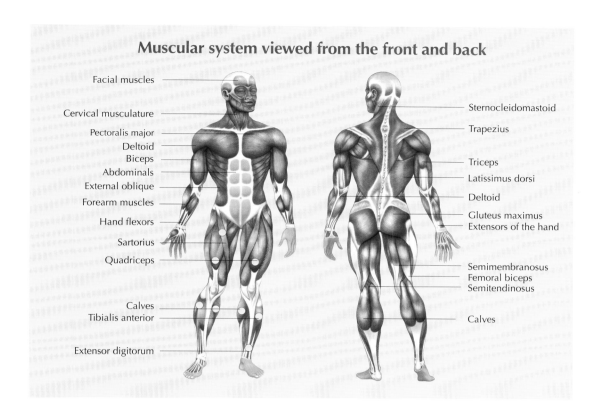

Muscular system viewed from the front and back

Facial muscles
Cervical musculature
Pectoralis major
Deltoid
Biceps
Abdominals
External oblique
Forearm muscles
Hand flexors
Sartorius
Quadriceps
Calves
Tibialis anterior
Extensor digitorum

Sternocleidomastoid
Trapezius
Triceps
Latissimus dorsi
Deltoid
Gluteus maximus
Extensors of the hand
Semimembranosus
Femoral biceps
Semitendinosus
Calves

The body is our vehicle with which we express what we feel. Holistic medicine knows that almost all disease and pain that occur in the body are due to psycho-emotive reasons; that is, the body somatizes emotional, energetic, and mental problems in specific areas, depending on the type of emotion. For example, in Traditional Chinese Medicine there are five emotions that affect five organs (see diagram below).

Knowing this gives us a great responsibility: maintaining our physical well-being by responding to the deeper aspects of our emotional and mental health. Practicing yoga with your partner helps you maintain an elevated level of well-being, energy, and health.

First, we have to get to know our body, since many people do not even know how many bones and muscles they have, or where their vital organs such as the liver are located.

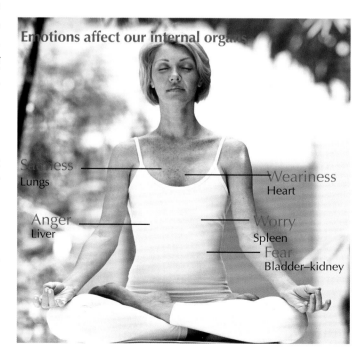

Emotions affect our internal organs

Sadness
Lungs

Anger
Liver

Weariness
Heart

Worry
Spleen

Fear
Bladder–kidney

Perfume of the divine
With each inhale, you breathe in God

The fragrance of practicing yoga with a partner translates into a delicate sense of well-being and elasticity that surrounds the body with a fine perfume.

By gaining a deeper understanding for our practice, and how it expresses the solar and lunar forces, we will feel as though we have crossed the threshold far beyond a simple combination of exercises.

Yoga is a science that emphasizes two energies: that of the Sun and that of the Moon, creating harmony and proper functioning of opposite pairs we have in the body: two cerebral hemispheres, two nostrils, two lungs, two kidneys, etc.

Bipolar forces let yogis enter into a current that illuminates the energy field, or aura, where they can perceive that there is greater universal unity.

Those who want to delve into this state will find a doorway to holistic perception of life, body, and emotions, traveling towards their inner world by closely studying their body language, following their heart and spirit.

Valuing the divinity that dwells in your partner—their heartbeat, mysterious energies of the human body, miles of veins—and valuing their company and the miracle of being alive is a sacred gift that comes from practicing sadhana.

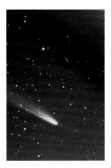

"He who knows the reality of the body knows the reality of the universe."

Tantric Principle

"The best protection against any disease is a noble mind."

PARACELSUS

Capturing the moment

Eastern disciplines such as Zen, Buddhism, tantra, and yoga have insisted on capturing the present.

The past brings back memories; the future, worry; and the present . . . is eternity! If we stop to reason we realize that there can be no point in time when the eternal is not present. If something is eternal, it is always, so your mind will cease to wander back and forth and start to focus on the now.

An important pillar of practicing yoga is breathing, which is not done yesterday or tomorrow; we breathe in the now and make a positive connection between our breath, our mind, and the present moment.

Satori in Zen, nirvana in Buddhism, or samadhi in yoga and tantra emphasize that this state comes from an instant of mindlessness without thoughts, worries, or ego, where mindfulness expands infinitely with the universal consciousness.

"The past brings back memories; the future, worry and anxiety. Whoever lives in the present is able to transcend time and remain eternal."

ESOTERIC PROVERB

Poses and counterposes

The spine is the axis of flexibility for all asanas. Therefore, whenever we backbend in certain poses, we need to compensate for such movement with two forward-bending poses.

The vertebrae acquire enormous flexibility and elasticity with practice, and it is very encouraging when you are able to see new results daily.

Practicing asanas with a partner lets you do a pose and its counterpose by taking turns. And since two poses can be done at a time, each partner gets to do many movements.

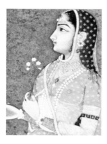

The fragrance of practicing yoga with a partner translates into a delicate sense of well-being.

Principles for practicing asanas

Each position requires following certain guidelines so that the physical, mental, and energetic changes can unfold properly.

1. Breathe slowly and consciously, most often through the nose.

2. Hold each position for at least thirty seconds to three minutes.

3. Do not ask too much of yourself, neither physically nor mentally.

4. Enjoy stretching without competing or wanting to "achieve" any idea of perfection.

5. Try to make slow and gentle movements at all times.

6. Do not practice asanas after eating; wait at least an hour.

7. Persevere; take it as a sacred ritual.

8. Rest your tongue against the roof of your mouth at all times.

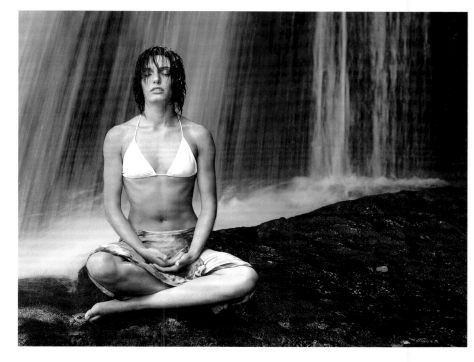

Questions about the practice
Yoga is very beneficial when it is done with a good guide

Fortunately for us, yoga has spread well throughout the West in its various forms, but some may still have questions about practicing with a partner.

• We are two older adults; can we do asanas with a partner?

Everyone's body is different. First you need to know how your spine is doing. Yoga works the spine and since it flexes the spine, one of its added benefits is that it fixes scoliosis, kyphosis, and lordosis.

Age is not an impediment as long as you respect each other's yin pace (slow and smooth); that is, go slowly at a pace that is adaptable for both people. Some asanas can be done more dynamically, such as standing poses, or by holding it for a certain number of breaths, such as seated poses.

Before starting your practice, remember that "a loving spirit never gets old." Be careful during your practice, bring awareness, and connect your consciousness, body, and breathing as if they were a single energy.

• I have been practicing yoga for two years, but my husband does not exercise and also smokes; can he participate?

My experience has taught me that women show more interest in yoga because their spiritual curiosity is greater. Most men are attached to the material, but some of them do like to take up yoga so if this is his case, there is no problem with him practicing with you; but be sure to guide him during the first weeks, let him know that he may experience "soreness," and reassure him that his body will become more flexible and gradually change.

It is important that the height and weight of both partners match up, and if he is overweight, he should go out for walks and adopt healthy eating habits (never going hungry) so his body will slim down.

"A spirit that loves never grows old."

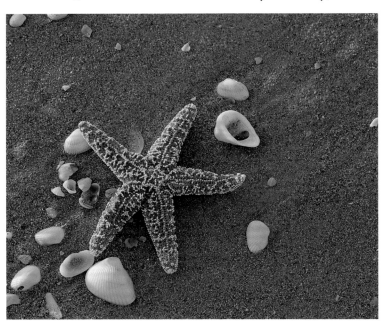

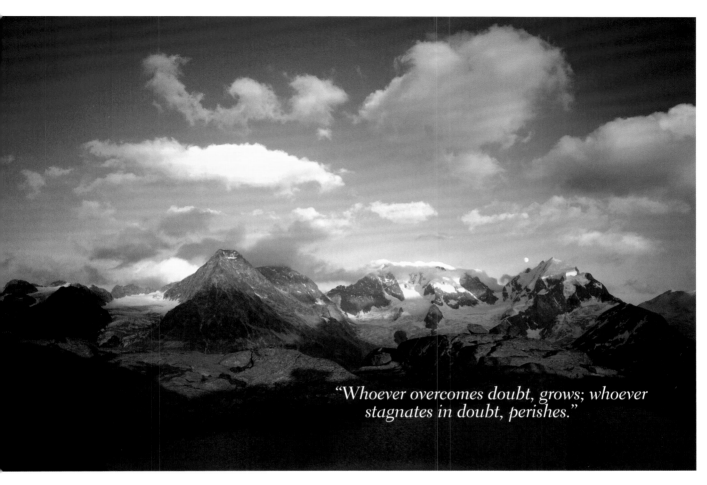

"Whoever overcomes doubt, grows; whoever stagnates in doubt, perishes."

Begin gradually and feel how your practice gives you pleasure from physical stretching and more communication due to your emotional openness.

Set your practice for a time when you know you will not be interrupted, and do not push your partner if he does not feel like doing it; the mind is lazy, but do not let laziness overcome you.

You could start by dancing as a warm-up. Regarding his smoking addiction, breathing exercises (pranayama) will purify his cells and feed his meridians with light so if his smoking is due to anxiety, he will become more relaxed.

Take notes on the different stretching exercises you do during the first class and compare them after a month. Motivate your partner whenever there is progress in his flexibility and consistency. You can give him a massage every time he practices during that first week and later massage each other as part of your practice.

• What do we need to practice yoga with a partner?
Willpower. Perseverance. Enjoyment. Consider it a sacred game. Intelligence. A comfortable and well-ventilated place. Also, avoid ingesting food for at least one hour prior to your practice.

Set your practice for a time when you will not be interrupted.

• We are two friends; can we practice even if we are of the same gender?

Of course. Yoga with a partner is the union of polarities, but all human beings are androgynous: our left half is feminine and our right half is male.

In each of you, one part will be more predominant. In addition, the connection and sisterhood between women is often stronger than the bond between man and woman. You can focus on practicing for the physical benefit without exploring your emotions deeply, but you will surely feel a strong sense of unity and communication, as sisters or lovers.

• I suffer from cancer; is it beneficial to practice with someone else?

As my friend Dr. Simón Mina, a holistic physician disciple of Dr. Hammer, said: "You can think of illness using your old pattern of thought that says that cancer equals death, or you can believe that your body is undergoing a healing process." What is yoga if not a path to good health? It is my wish that you practice to rejuvenate and brighten your cells, boost your energy, release negative thoughts, connect with your soul (which uses the language of healing) and to let a new healthy, natural, and clean you be born within. Listen to classical music during your practice, let Pavarotti or Vivaldi enhance your

Yoga with a partner is the union of polarities, but all human beings are androgynous.

asanas, laugh at your organs, glands, and start an internal revolution!

By practicing with another person you will benefit from an exchange of energy, which will increase your vitality. Respect your own pace and mind your breathing rhythm.

Remember that you are in the process of healing and that practicing yoga can really help you in this process. Stay strong!

• We are a young couple who never practice any sports, except for a little aerobics. What can we get out of practicing yoga with a partner?

It is great to start practicing while you are young so you can continue doing it throughout your lifetime.

Young cells and atoms, whose center is light, capture light energy that gives life for therapeutic purposes. Practicing yoga with a partner can help stop the aging process and prolong youth because it prevents cells from getting filled with toxins and because we eat light and energetic sattvic food and practice asanas and pranayama.

It is important for you to figure out what you will do with so much energy, because when we are young our vitality is at its highest and if we are not mindfully guided we could become very angry, aggressive, or anxious. Seek an outlet of art, love, and creativity where you can direct this vital flow.

If it is not properly channeled, your energy flow can cause discomfort, pain, and even irritability.

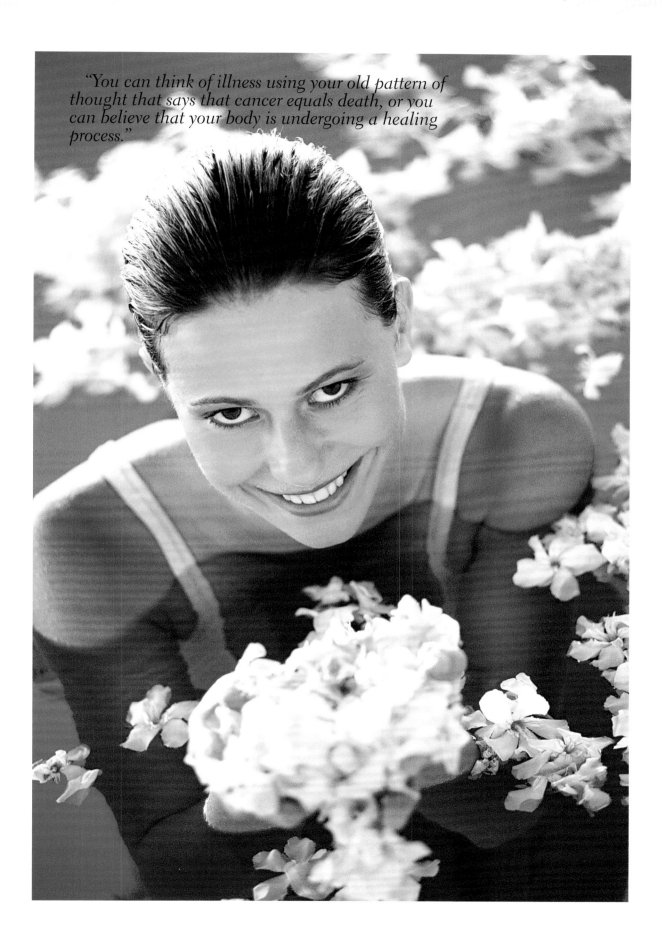

"You can think of illness using your old pattern of thought that says that cancer equals death, or you can believe that your body is undergoing a healing process."

Pranayamas. Pranic food
"For yogis, breathing is a science"

Pranayamas are special exercises to get more prana through breathing techniques. Prana, as I stated, is in the air, it contains neither oxygen nor nitrogen, but rather negative ions: small packets of pure energy.

We breathe 15 to 18 times a minute, 21,600 times a day. Our lungs have the ability to take in five liters of air; it is our first food. As the old adage goes, "He who learns to breathe learns to live."

Pranayama is a divine tool, a magical gift for humans to increase their energy, expand their consciousness, and enter into a meditative state where existence is perceived as light, consciousness, and magic.

The fundamental law of prana is that it responds to thought; that is, visualization and intention is paramount when it comes to applying it for more energy. Wherever your thought is, that is where your energy will be as well.

> "There is no greater power food on Earth than breathing techniques."
>
> YOGIC PRINCIPLE

Abdominal breathing

While lying in shavasana, let your abdomen inflate and deflate. It will rise and fall like ocean waves. Only the lower part is used during this breath.

Benefits

Fills your solar plexus with prana.
Lets you enter into a state of relaxation.
Relaxes your mind as though you were a baby.
Oxygenates your stomach.

Duration. 5 to 30 minutes.

Ujjayi Breath

Sit in vajrasana or siddhasana; with your mouth closed, inhale the outside air through your nostrils and exhale freely. You will make a soft, audible sound.

Benefits

Completely fills the lungs with prana.
Activates your energy circuit.
Prepares you for meditation.
Releases dormant energies.
Enlarges your lung capacity.

Duration. 5 to 10 minutes.

Pranayamas have three phases

1. **Puraka.** Inhalation phase. The lungs are filled.
2. **Kumbhaka.** Breath retention phase. During these few seconds inhaled prana can be stored.
3. **Rechaka.** Exhalation phase. After retaining its energy, freely exhale out all the air.

Alternate breathing

With a straight back, use your right thumb to cover your right nostril and inhale through the left nostril. Then use your left ring finger to cover your left nostril and exhale through the right nostril. Then inhale through the right nostril while covering your left nostril and exhale through the left nostril. This is one cycle.

Benefits

Cleanses the ida and pingala nadis.
Lets energy flow stronger.
Prepares you for dynamic or deep breathing.
Brings energy and oxygen to the two brain hemispheres, thus balancing its functions.
Duration. 7 full cycles.

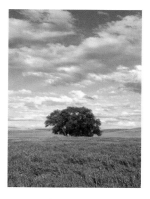

"He who learns to breathe learns to live."

How to do pranayama breathing

- Sit comfortably in vajrasana or siddhasana. It is important to keep your back completely straight, but if you are still not very flexible you can sit in a chair.
- Clear your mind of any worry or anxiety. Begin your pranayama exercises with a calm mind.
- During the kumbhaka (the re-tention), mentally repeat the mantra "Om," the primordial sacred sound.
- As you retain air, practice doing bandhas or body locks to store energy within and enhance your chakras.
- Do not force the lungs, especially during the retention stage.
- Visualize at all times divine light entering with each breath and how waste and toxins are removed with each exhalation.
- Focus your mind on the present through your breathing.

It is important to note that when your breathing rate changes, your emotional and mental state also changes.
- After each pranayama session, leave your energy in the chakra that most needs it. Prana is usually left in the manipura or anahatta chakra.
- Feel how your physical and energetic bodies, as well as your mind and spirit, make contact with the life principle of all beings. Let yourself be filled with electromagnetism.
- The best time for pranayama is between three and seven in the morning, when yang energy is emerging strongly. If you cannot do it in the morning, then noon and sunset are the best.
- Rest your tongue against the roof of the mouth to activate the nadis.

- Pranayama should not be done by pregnant women, people with recent heart surgery, hypertension, fever, or hemorrhage.

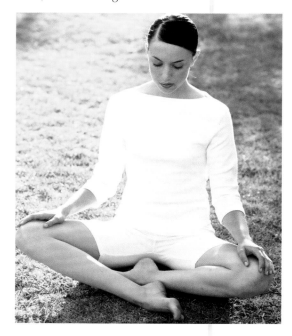

Bellows breath

Sit with your back straight, inhale, and exhale vigorously through both nostrils using short and dynamic breaths.

Benefits

Cleanses the nostrils.
Prevents colds.
Increases body heat.
Activates kundalini.
Raises awareness.
Oxygenates the brain.
Energizes the chakras.
Purifies the lungs.
Prevents and cures phlegm.
Activates energy in all its functions, especially sexual and intellectual energy.
Provides self-esteem, strong willpower, and inner joy.

Duration. Three sets of 30 breaths with three full breaths, and three bandhas between sets.

By increasing your daily practice, after a month you can increase it to five series of fifty breaths. Inhalation and exhalation count as one breath.

Full breath

This is quintessential yogi breathing. It consists of completing three stages of breathing: low or abdominal phase, middle or lung phase, and high or subclavian phase. To do so, slowly inhale through the nose and sink in your abdomen, inflate the chest and slightly raise your shoulders. Exhalation is done in reverse, from the top to the middle ending at the

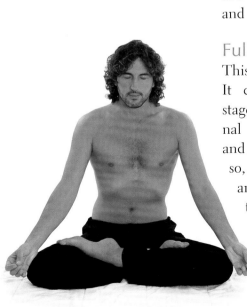

bottom, completely emptying your lungs.

Benefits

Increases breathing capacity.
Prevents and cures asthma.
Benefits pranic currents through the nadi, in particular sushumna, ida, and pingala.
Activates the seven chakras.
Aligns the spine.
Provides a sense of inner unity, and luminous energy expansion of your consciousness.

Duration. 5 to 20 minutes.

Sitali Breath

Inhale through the mouth with pursed lips while sticking out your tongue, and then slowly fill your stomach. Hold it briefly. Then exhale through both nostrils.

Benefits

Eliminates indigestion.
Refreshes the body.
Purifies the lungs and eliminates phlegm.
Protects from bile disorders.

Duration. 3 to 7 minutes.

Kapalabhati Breath

("Kapala" = skull; "bhati" = shine, clean)

Inhale (puraka) for twice as long as you energetically exhale (rechaka).

Benefits

Cleanses and purifies the lungs.
Charges the solar plexus with prana.
Stimulates circulation and throat.

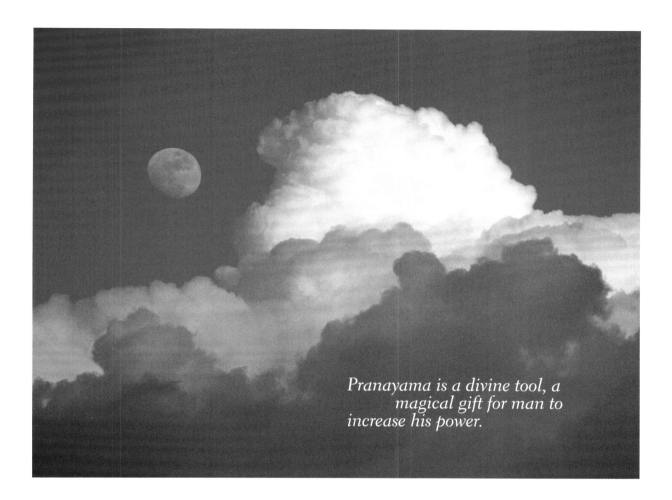

Pranayama is a divine tool, a magical gift for man to increase his power.

Increases body heat.

Oxygenates the blood.

Activates the chakras.

Strengthens abdominal muscles.

Improves digestion.

Tones the nervous system.

During inhalation brain volume decreases and during exhalation it increases.

Massages and cleanses the brain.

Revitalizes brain cells, activating the pineal and pituitary glands.

Eliminates fatigue and toxins.

Removes lactic acid.

Combats asthma.

Refreshes the eyes.

Activates Ajna and Sahasrara Chakras.

Prepares the mind for meditation.

Works on kundalini.

We bring in more oxygen and eliminate carbon dioxide.

It is different from "Bastrika" or "bellows" in that Kapalabhati puts more emphasis on exhalation, while for "Bastrika" it is done an equal amount of times.

By holding air in our lungs, we can hold prana longer within and close our bandhas.

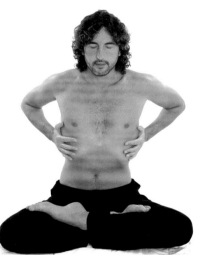

Duration. Start with two sets of forty breaths (inhalation and exhalation count as one), until you can do three sets of 120 with constant practice. Hold your breath for five to ten seconds at intervals between sets.

Circular breathing

Tantric circle or circular breathing is a breathing meditation that tends to dissolve the boundaries of the body and awaken energy sensitivity.

It is breathing that connects inhalation and exhalation without any space in between. Inhaling and exhaling is done in the same amount of time.

It can be done alone or with a partner, forming an even stronger bond between the two.

Benefits

Awakens a sense of physical and spiritual unity.

Activates energy through the meridians.

Expands the boundaries of the mind.

Prepares you for entering into a deep meditative state.

Gives peace and quiet.

Lets you feel energy in the second body and fill yourself with "pure consciousness."

Duration. 20 to 40 minutes.

Have energy every day

In the morning

1. Polarized breath: 7 cycles
2. Recharging breath: 10 minutes
3. Full breath: 7 cycles
4. Mahabhandas: 7 breaths with the three bandhas
5. Abdominal breath: 3 minutes

Total time: 25 to 30 minutes.

At sunset

1. Cleansing breath: ten minutes
2. Chakras breath: seven cycles for each
3. Circular breath, alone or with a partner: fifteen minutes
4. Abdominal breath: ten minutes

Total time: about 45 minutes.

Pranayamas are very strong, so start slowly, feeling the reactions that your body and psyche experience.

Remember that in nature nothing blooms overnight. And also remember that all energy is neutral: fire can warm you up in the winter but in excess it can burn a forest. Similarly, pranayamas are useful to the extent that they fill you with vitality.

It is important for you to have an intended use for the energy you are awakening; channel it toward something creative. If you follow these steps, you will awaken your own inner teacher. Those who are suffering from high blood pressure, eye problems, or recent heart surgery must abstain from practicing kapalabhati, recharging, and chakras pranayama; but for everyone else, these practices are harmless.

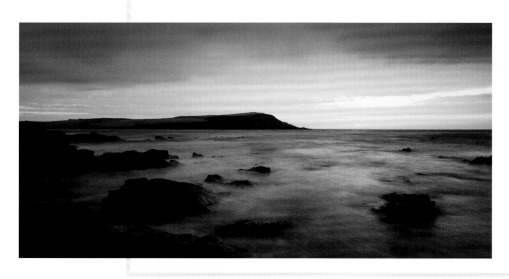

Cleansing breath

With this practice the body is cleansed of stale or stagnant energy, and it recharges with prana. It is very useful when you have been among people with negative or dense energy. In fact, contamination is inevitable in our everyday living environment; ranging from household appliances to smoke from factories or cars.

Inhale through your nose and exhale through the mouth. For best results do this in shavasana, lying on your back.

Benefits
Cleanses the meridians.
Cleanses and unlocks the solar plexus, where heavy energy tends to stagnate.
Recharges your chakras with prana.

Duration. 10 to 20 minutes.

Recharging breath

Every morning, practice this technique just as you would recharge your cell phone's battery.

Stand with your legs shoulder width apart, take short and forceful breaths, like bellows, and shake your head, shoulders, arms, and hands as though you were covered in flour and needed to shake it off.

Do it quickly and make sure that you do not interrupt your breathing. Stop after five or ten minutes and do seven complete breaths as you envision your whole body being wrapped in light. You will have a lot of energy throughout the day.

It is a natural vitamin that increases blood flow to the brain.

Benefits
Energizes the nervous system.
Powerfully activates the chakras and kundalini.
Cleanses the nostrils.
Fresh blood and prana flow to the brain.
Improves memory.
Puts you in a good mood.
Lets your physical body stay healthy and strong without getting tired.

Duration. 3 to 5 minutes the first week, every day. Then increase it to ten minutes at most.

Chakras breath

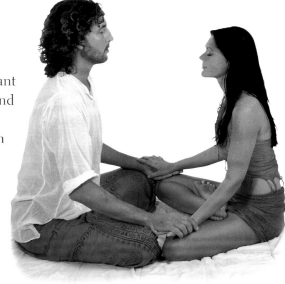

This is an important exercise to cleanse and activate the chakras.

Inhale through your nose and exhale through the mouth while visualizing each chakra and its circular shape with its own color. Do seven slow, deep, conscious breaths for each chakra. Follow the order of the chakras as you visualize red, orange, yellow, green, blue, white, and violet. Move your sexual energy towards the brahamaranda, the seat of the divine on top of your head.

Benefits
Activates, purifies, and cleanses all chakras and elevates your kundalini.

Duration. 20 to 45 minutes. Do three cycles, from the first to the seventh chakra.

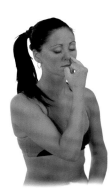

Surya breath: solar breathing

Covering your left nostril, inhale and exhale using only your right nostril. This nostril is usually more active on Mondays, Tuesdays, and Saturdays, and more intensely during the dark half of the lunar cycle when the moon is waning and new.

Benefits
Activates the left hemisphere of the brain.
Warms up your physical body.

Duration. 7 cycles.

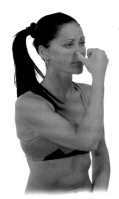

Chandra Breath: lunar breathing

Covering your right nostril, inhale and exhale only using your left nostril. Normal breathing through this nostril flows stronger on Wednesdays, Thursdays, Fridays, and Sundays, and it is enhanced when the moon shines brightly.

Benefits
Activates the right hemisphere of the brain. Refreshes the body, so it is good to do it in the summer.
It has a positive effect on the sympathetic nervous system and our bodily functions.
Activates Shakti, the feminine principle.

Duration. 7 cycles.

Shiva-Shakti Pranayama: great tantric breathing

Sitting face-to-face, in diamond or half lotus pose, rest your forehead against your partner's and connect using your third eye, and breathe as follows: Shiva (man) exhales through the nose while Shakti (woman) inhales his exhaled air; then she exhales and he inhales.

Universal breath

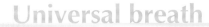

Seated at arm's length, fold your legs in half lotus or lotus, place your hands at the center of your chest in pranava mudra, and exhale all the air out while making two circles with your arms. Inhale and make two circles with your hands, this time towards the center of your chest, and bring them together. Then stop and meditate while visualizing the green color of that chakra.

Benefits
Connects with the heart.
Calms the mind.

Brings energy to the fourth chakra.
Strengthens your relationship.

Duration.
At least 10 minutes.

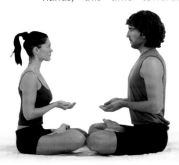
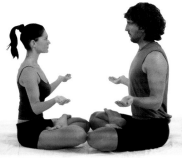
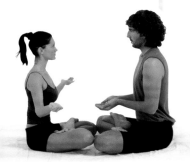

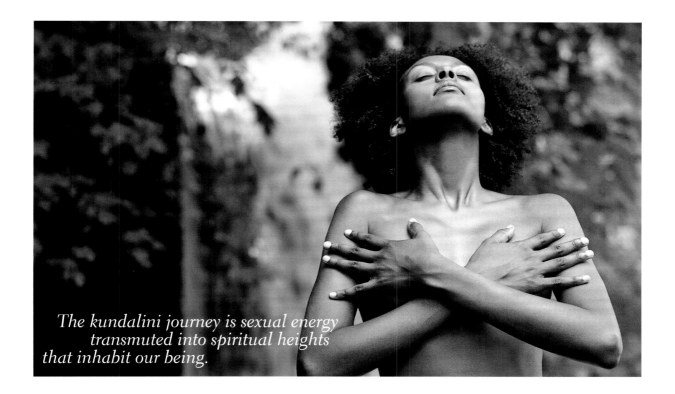

The kundalini journey is sexual energy transmuted into spiritual heights that inhabit our being.

Benefits

Powerfully connects your energy fields.
Merges souls beyond the boundaries of individuality.
Shares the miracle of breathing.
Awakens telepathy.
Recycles energy by joining the yin and yang, negative and positive.
Generates electricity and magnetism, allowing for more light in the cells and in all areas of emotional life.

Duration: one cycle for at least 10 minutes.

Kundalini voyage

This is the maximum energy path that we can reach as human beings: bringing energy up from the sacrum (sacred) to the head (crown). This "sacred crown" is the arrival of sexual energy transmuted into spiritual heights that inhabit our being.

This breathing/meditation enables us to become familiar with sensing this energy. Sitting in half lotus, with your back against your partner's, inhale and exhale while visualizing how energy moves up from one chakra to the next. You can imagine the colors of each chakra to intensify their effect.

Benefits

Elevates your energy, psyche, and vitality.
Grants you access to every inner realm: animal, human, and divine.
Merges energies.
Transmutes sexual energy into spiritual energy without repression.
It is an ideal bridge for bonding your bodies and souls deeply before lovemaking.

This breathing/ meditation enables us to become familiar with sensing this energy.

Warm up your body with dance

"By dancing, you move in harmony with the whole Universe"

By dancing in my tantra and yoga courses, I look primarily to rid the body of tension and repression. By letting your body loose you release energy. Music, rhythm, and cleansing breath will make our emotions and mind loosen their grip over us.

The enormous power, openness, and inner joy that is experienced in ethnic dances are like a gardener watering flowers. You feel ancestral, natural, and connected to life.

Heat and energy awakened by dance is great for your physical body and they are perfect as warm-up exercise so you can correctly practice asanas.

According to yoga, we can be fluid and flexible like a river, and dancing with meditative awareness can make a profound change in our internal state.

Stiffness equals death; hence flexibility and lightness that dancing gives us is like an energy injection and a treat for our body and soul.

Many people feel transported to a different place when they dance. And there is an explanation for this: if you forget about schedules, routine, concerns, and constraints, what else is left? By nurturing your own intrinsic nature—power, joy, peace of mind, sensuality—dancing brings you back to your natural state, tears down barriers created by the ego, and repays debt with affection.

Whenever you dance with drums or tribal music, feel how your chest opens with every breath, how your cells and organs dance as well, how your blood flows, how your muscles warm up, and how your soul flows. Breathing is the fuel that ignites energy. Inhale through your nose and exhale through your mouth at all times and stay conscious and alert to how energy rises through the chakras.

Kundalini is also activated through dancing: serpentine fire spreads and feeds each of your energy centers.

Dancing is a form of meditation, and it becomes even more powerful when you practice it with a partner because you get to exchange your energy field and create a balance between yin and yang.

When you dance with different partners, there is a powerful enrichment; you become more aware of your energy and you will get in touch with the innate wisdom of your body and soul, not your mind.

Dancing clears up any barriers that your bad habits or conditioning have created, opens up emotions, and releases tension.

Music, rhythms, and cleansing breath will make your emotions and mind lose control.

Your body gets unblocked, especially in the sexual area and head, and you will experience joy, mental silence, and synchrony with the universe and all creation. You will feel relief from physical pain, back pain, and emotional pain, and a real liberating catharsis.

"Conscious dance takes us back to our human nature."

Breathe energy and feel freedom in your heart

As you practice asanas, it is essential that you breathe and feel.

Through breathing, you will get new energy and eliminate dormant tensions and energies. Practice breathing, meditative awareness, and sensitivity so you can get the most from dancing.

Tips for dancing
1. Breathe consciously.
2. Disconnect the mind.
3. Set your entire body free, especially the pelvis, neck, and head.
4. Get your whole being involved in the dance.
5. Feel the kundalini and elevate it.
6. Be open to experiencing the divine.
7. Let movement take you to the stillness and let music transport you into silence.

When you dance, you use breathing as a means to ignite your inner spirit. Just as air fuels fire, conscious breathing fuels your spirit.

Breathing brings you into the present moment without letting your mind interfere with thoughts or future worry; that is why it is an important element in our relationship with the eternal.

Benefits of dancing

Benefits of dancing before practicing asanas:

- Balances your emotions
- Strengthens your self-confidence
- Softens facial features and body expression
- Relieves deep tensions
- Brings joy and well-being to your everyday life

- Raises kundalini
- Corrects poor physical posture, eliminating back pain and shoulder tension
- Unblocks the genital area, letting you enjoy sex even more
- Helps during labor and menstruation
- Awakens your spiritual power
- Increases creativity and enthusiasm

- Quickly quiets your mind
- Deepens your breathing
- Creates a connection between you and Creation
- Puts you in sync with intuition, freedom, and joy
- Strengthens your soul

Principles for asanas

"By practicing asanas, you connect with your inner God"

Each asana lets us feel flexibility, strength, openness, serenity, cold, heat, tingling, blood circulation, and energy . . . Our body is alive!

Spinal column

The spinal column is the tree of life. From the sacrum (sacred) to the atlas bone we have thirty-three vertebrae surrounded in mystery.

From the neck to the dorsal, lumbar, and sacral area, health depends on having flexible spinal discs, elasticity, firmness, and correct posture. So healthy longevity consists of keeping our spine youthful through yoga practice, a discipline that is primarily responsible for lending us flexibility. To maintain your energy, your chakras will turn on and activate your consciousness, which may be dormant or blocked. Expansive poses, for example backbends, allow for greater opening of the fourth chakra (responsible for developing higher emotions), so by practicing them you will get a clear sense of openness, feel your chest open, and breathe much more freely (linked to emotions).

Regular practice will also help you address physical spinal problems such as scoliosis, cervical and lumbar lordosis, and thoracic kyphosis.

The spine is the tree of life.

Each pose is designed to stimulate your bones and your energy level and let your spine come to its correct position.

The pressure of life goes straight to the spine, just as fear of death affects the knees, and fear of being yourself affects the feet, so by correcting the posture of your spine you will experience changes at the psychological level, such as reevaluating your life's purpose and increasing your self-esteem, as well as making your body more flexible and strong like a tree that withstands a difficult storm.

Breathing

It is the cornerstone for practicing yoga. Most positions are held while mentally counting a number of breaths for the duration of each asana.

Breathing equals life and energy, so by keeping a certain pace in their breathing, yogis are able to connect through a silent and shared language that goes beyond intellect. Breathing can change your energy level, feelings, and mental state, because emotions and thoughts are determined by the rhythm of your breathing.

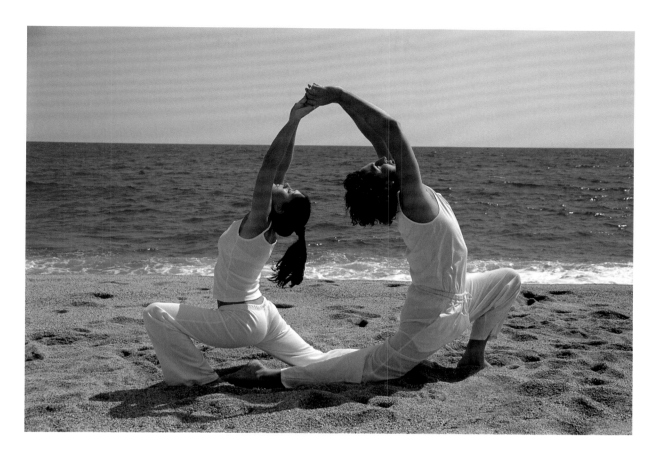

For instance, if you are feeling anxious or angry you will take very quick and shallow breaths. However, in stillness, peace, and harmony, your breathing will be slow and methodical.

Yoga emphasizes this important aspect that will largely determine the success of your practice.

Permanence

The element of permanence in each asana is determined by its degree of difficulty.

Some asanas are done vigorously, while others requiring a greater amount of stillness are combined with slow and rhythmic breathing.

Stay in each pose as you experience pleasure at all times without pain or exertion.

Try to vary the duration of each exercise depending on your individual needs and the pleasure you feel with each asana.

Comfort

There are varying degrees of flexibility.

Through proper breathing, support, and harmony with a partner, we get to comfortable asanas that encourage us to continue with our practice, and we tend to persist in activities that we find beneficial.

Give yourself the gift of setting aside some time each day to practice yoga and relax.

Through proper breathing, support, and harmony with a partner, we get to comfortable asanas that encourage us to continue with our practice.

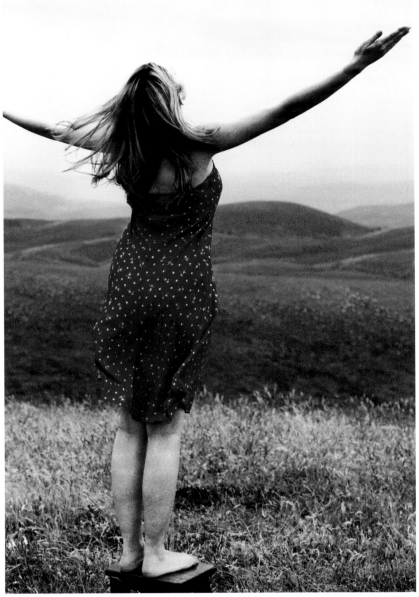

movements, duration, and alignment with the required amount of support.

Perception of energy

"Energy is every phenomenon that produces movement."

Yoga with a partner, tantra, and other paths toward personal growth seek to capture a greater flow of energy and, most importantly, close any "leakage" where energy gets lost. This increases our vitality and lets us make better use of this precious gift (which is a form of Jnana yoga, or "knowledge used wisely").

On the other hand, certain activities and people can absorb your energy.

It would help for you to come up with your own list:

1. Ten people or activities that take away your energy.
2. Ten activities that you like to do but keep postponing.
3. Your bad habits.
4. Little annoyances that you tolerate.
5. Everything you "should have done."

Take all the time you need to make this list. You will find decisive answers so that the energy you "create" and accumulate by practicing yoga does not escape in ways that do not contribute to growth or creativity.

Many times, your quality of life will suffer through unconscious leakage of vitality due to the things you "should do" and spending time with people whose energy is extremely negative.

Body weight

To prevent injuries you must know whether there is a marked difference in weight between you and your partner. It is also important that neither partner places all his or her weight onto the other person.

Supporting the body becomes progressively easier as the partners synchronize their breathing and increase their communication.

To successfully do each asana, follow the instructions for

With the intention of avoiding losing so much energy and in order to live many years, yogis invented a method of rhythmic breathing. Just as our blood system absorbs oxygen, the nervous system and chakras absorb prana and use it to process our desires, impulses, actions, thoughts, feelings, etc. Regulating breathing and yoga asanas with a partner allows us to build up more energy in the brain and nervous system. This energy is then ready for our use when we need it most. Of course this gets better with practice. Ancient mystics and advanced yogis have given us the key to practice using our spirituality daily. Also keep in mind that every organ in our body depends on the nervous system and it is nourished by prana energy from the Sun that spreads through the universe. Our organs could not function without this energy; and that is important, right?

Prana is not only nutrition, but it also transmits energy to the nervous system and it magnetizes the body and aura. Practicing yoga techniques with a partner can easily help us attain this magnetization.

Thus, couples that practice yoga together are distinguished by their vitality, magnetism, and energy. Listlessness, pallor, and coldness disappear from their lives because they eliminate eighty percent of all toxins and their mental, psychological, physical, energetic, and emotional states get cleansed. In fact, yoga is purification at all levels.

Yoga is holistic purification.

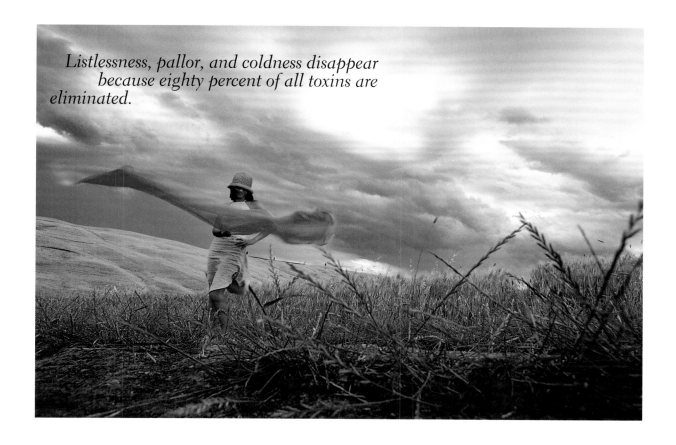

Listlessness, pallor, and coldness disappear because eighty percent of all toxins are eliminated.

Chakras Overview

Chakras	Desire it generates	Plexus	Glands	Systems and organs	Elements	Senses	Function	Mantra	Body	Color
Sahasrara	Spiritual desire	Coronary	Pineal	Mind, spiritual life	–	–	Communication with the transcendent	–	Spiritual	Purple Golden
Ajna	Desire for knowledge	Frontal	Pituitary	Mind, base of skull, brain stem, cerebellum, higher mind	Manas (mental abilities)	Internal	Clairvoyance	Om	Higher mind	White
Vishuddha	Desire to create and express	Throat	Thyroid	Respiratory, voice, neck, face, lips, ears, eyes, words, eyebrows, muscles, fingers, five senses	Ether	Hearing	Intellect	Ham	Intellectual or inferior mind	Blue
Anahata	Desire to love and be loved	Cardiac	Thymus	Circulatory, chest, upper thoracic spine, arms, palms of the hands	Air	Touch	Affection	Yam	Affective or higher emotions	Green
Manipura	Desire for food	Solar	Pancreas	Digestive, upper abdomen, lower spine, stomach, liver, gallbladder, pancreas	Fire	Sight	Convergence of energy	Ram	Emotional	Yellow
Svadhish-thana	Sexual desire	Splenic	Adrenal	Knees, urogenital, lumbosacral spine, hips, pelvis, arch of the foot	Water	Taste	Instincts	Vam	Energetic or vital	Orange
Muladhara	Earthly survival	Coccygeal	Sexual	Urogenital, legs, feet	Earth	Smell	Basis for kundalini	Lam	Organic or dense	Red

Petals	Geometric figure	Meditation achievements	Location	Balanced emotional and psychological qualities	Unbalanced emotional and psychological qualities	Awareness level	Physical conditions associated with unbalance	Corresponding poses
1000	△	Integration and connection to the transcendent spiritual realm	Crown (release)	Universal energy and cosmic consciousness, cosmic love, inspiration, enlightenment	Depression, confinement, narrow-mindedness, dementia, psychosis, worry	Higher emotions, spiritual will	Brain tumor, cranial pressure	
2	○	Intuition and control of the body and spirit	Third eye. (visualization)	Intellectual and psychic abilities, visualization, imagination, projection, perception	Difficulty focusing on life, schizophrenia, isolation, intellectual stagnation	Concrete thoughts, higher mind	Headaches, fuzzy thinking	
16	○	Understanding and speaking power	Throat (vocal expression)	Communication, expression, creativity, inspiration, interaction	Stagnation, obsession, lack of expression	Concrete thoughts	Sore throat, vocal cord problems, colds, thyroid problems	
12	⬡ ✡	Devotion and knowledge	Center of the chest	Compassion, acceptance, love, accomplishment	Insensitivity, emotionally closed, passivity, sadness	Concrete emotions, personal, higher emotions	Cardiovascular problems, arthritis, respiratory problems, stroke, hypertension	
10	☾	Compassion and fitness	Between the base of the sternum and the navel (personal power)	Personal power, motivation, decisions, willpower, self-image	Inefficiency, greed, doubt, anger, guilt	Vital instinct	Ulcer, jaundice, hepatitis, hypoglycemia, gallstones	
6	△	Control of apana (energy for eliminating waste)	Halfway between the navel and pubis (sexuality, creativity, energy deposit)	Patience, endurance, self-confidence, well-being	Frustration, affection, anxiety, fear	Vital instinct	Sexual impotence, diabetes, hypersexuality, kidney and bladder problems	
4	□	Sublimation of physical nature	Base of the spine (stability)	Security, stability, sense of preservation	Self-indulgence, selfishness, insecurity, instability, grief, depression	Physical	Hemorrhoids, constipation, sciatica, prostate problems	

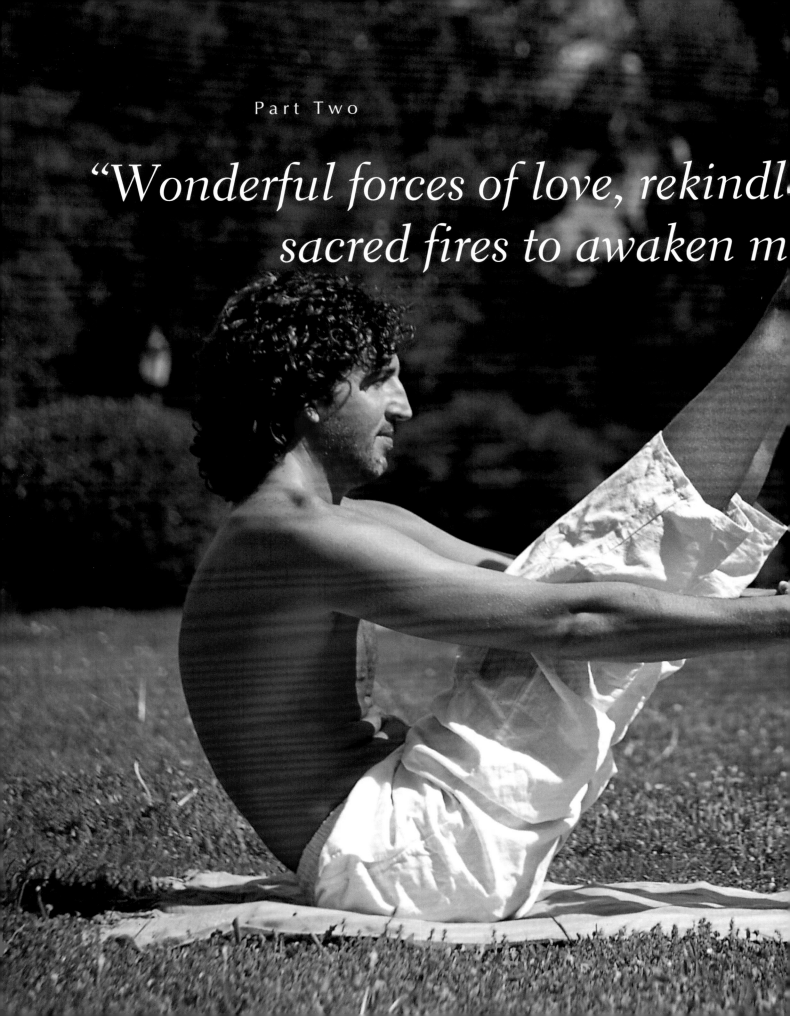

Part Two

"Wonderful forces of love, rekindl
sacred fires to awaken m

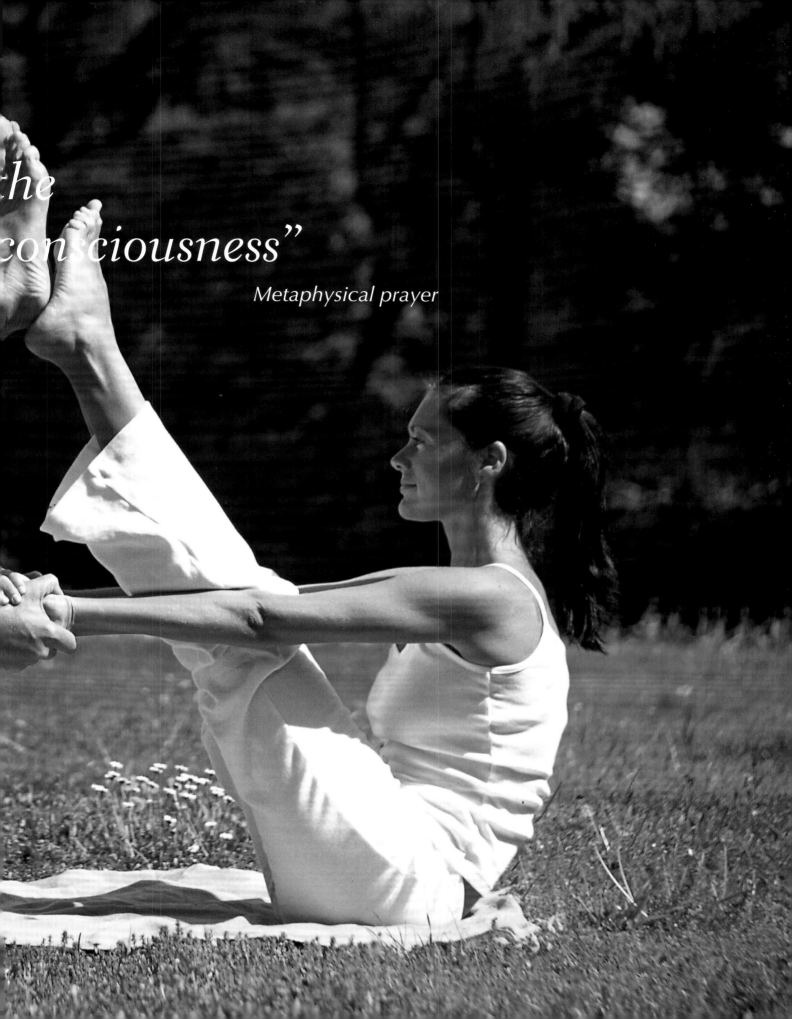

...the

"...consciousness"

Metaphysical prayer

Instructions

Practice, benefits, and categories

Asanas, or psychotherapeutic yoga poses, are an art in and of themselves and there is a long history of yogis who have attained enlightenment and physical well-being by consciously working with them.

Like any art, it takes practice, perseverance, and discipline. Yoga is not a hobby but a laboratory where we can learn about ourselves. It is the possibility of connecting with unknown spaces of the body, mind, and spirit, providing countless benefits to its practitioners.

Each type of asana works using the backbone and the whole body.

A full session of yoga must have a balanced number of asanas, but it can also be structured for specific areas of the body, using vinyasas for example, which is a pose developed in all its possible variants.

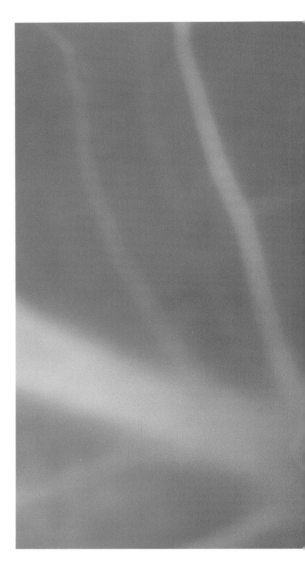

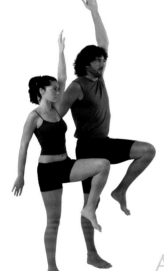

Asanas by category

1. Standing poses

2. Meditation poses

3. Forward-bending poses

4. Back-bending poses

5. Balancing poses

6. Strengthening poses

7. Inversions

8. Twists

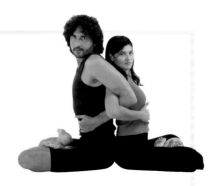

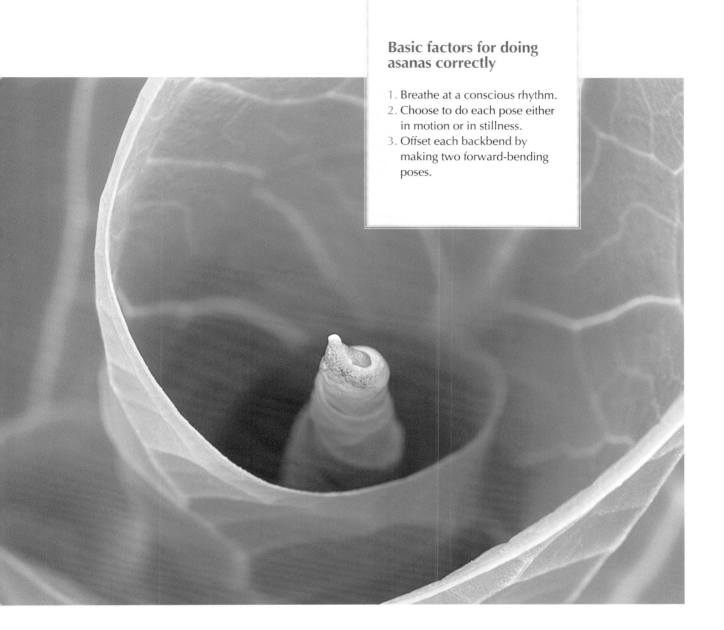

Basic factors for doing asanas correctly

1. Breathe at a conscious rhythm.
2. Choose to do each pose either in motion or in stillness.
3. Offset each backbend by making two forward-bending poses.

Energy exchange in yoga with your partner

Working with hatha and kundalini yoga brings your chakras together, which greatly enhances your energy exchange and synchronization. By regularly practicing asanas, you and your partner will awaken your many siddhis or extrasensory powers, such as telepathy (knowing what the other person will say or speaking at the same time), perceptions, intuition, or clairvoyance, which means that your higher chakras are opening.

Bioenergy currents that flow whenever you practice asanas are comprehensive nourishment: physical, loving, and existential communication between lovers.

Dynamic asanas

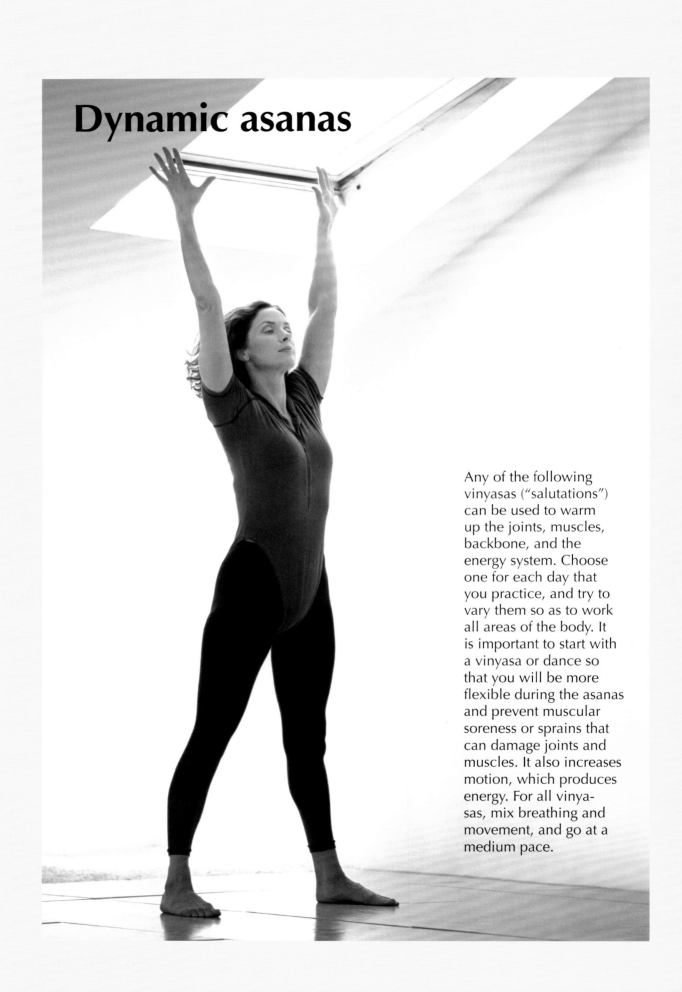

Any of the following vinyasas ("salutations") can be used to warm up the joints, muscles, backbone, and the energy system. Choose one for each day that you practice, and try to vary them so as to work all areas of the body. It is important to start with a vinyasa or dance so that you will be more flexible during the asanas and prevent muscular soreness or sprains that can damage joints and muscles. It also increases motion, which produces energy. For all vinyasas, mix breathing and movement, and go at a medium pace.

The following illustrations show
WARM-UP MOVEMENTS:

Balancing movement
Powerful posture
Extensive Yab-Yum
Bend and expand the spine

The CAT POSE sequence is also shown.

Warm-up movements
Activate the entire body and force of energy

1. Balancing Movement

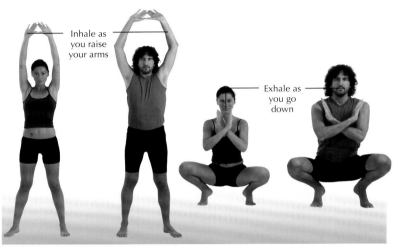

Inhale as you raise your arms

Exhale as you go down

Benefits
- Mobilizes energy and circulates blood throughout the body.
- Generates heat, so it is useful as a warm-up before doing asanas.
- Strengthens the knees.
- Increases your breathing capacity and your control over it.

Duration
Repeat 12 to 20 times.

1 Standing next to each other, 3 feet (one meter) apart, open your legs and stretch your arms as you deeply inhale.

2 Flex your legs and slowly crouch down. At the same time, cross your hands over your chest and exhale all the air.

2. Powerful Posture

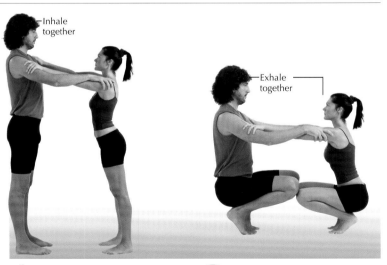

Inhale together

Exhale together

Benefits
- Increases leg strength and improves knee joints.
- Strengthens the heart.

Duration
15 to 25 breaths.

1 Stand face-to-face and spread your legs, stretch your arms, and place your hands on your partner's shoulders. Look into each other's eyes and inhale deeply before descending.

2 Bend your legs and slowly go down until you squat. Keep your back straight and exhale all the air.

3. Extensive Yab-Yum

This Tantric asana forms a circle of energy between both polarities.

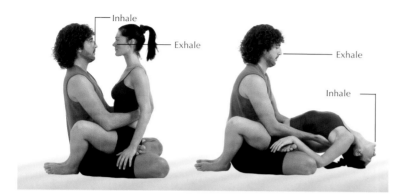

Inhale

Exhale

Exhale

Inhale

1 The man sits cross-legged in any of its variant poses. The woman sits on top of him with her legs spread open and uses her feet to press behind his sacrum. The man strongly holds her body at the waist and interlaces his fingers behind her back.

2 The woman lets herself fall back until she has completely stretched her spine and chest. She then exhales all the air and comes up very slowly to avoid getting dizzy.

Benefits
- Mobilizes energy and circulation.
- Opens the chest, the fourth and fifth chakras.
- Creates trusting bond.
- Opens emotions.
- Increases breathing capacity.
- Improves the functioning of the thyroid, pineal, and pituitary glands.
- Strengthens and rejuvenates the spine.

Duration
4 to 12 breaths.

4. Bend and expand the spine

Sitting face-to-face in a diamond pose, keep your back upright and place your hands on your thighs.

Benefits
- Rejuvenates the entire backbone, from the sacrum to the neck.
- Increases breathing capacity.
- Moves energy through the central channel or sushumna.

Duration
10 to 20 breaths in slow motion. You can increase the pace of movement and respiratory rate up to sixty breaths, as with bellows breath.

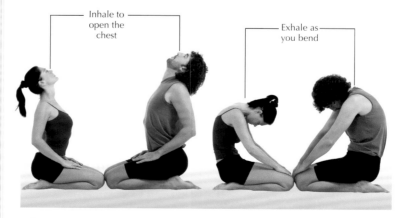

Inhale to open the chest

Exhale as you bend

1 Inhale as you bend back your spine and head, and expand your chest.

2 Exhale all the air while the spine curves inward, like the shell of a turtle.

Cat Pose
Gendrasa namaskar

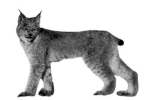

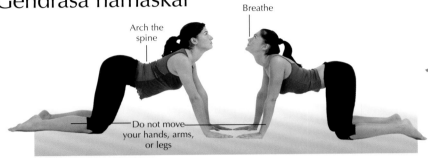

Arch the spine

Breathe

Do not move your hands, arms, or legs

1 Inhale and arch all your vertebrae.

Exhale as you bend forward

2 Only move the spine.

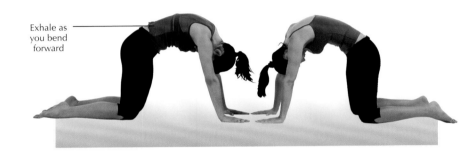

Inhale and stretch one leg

3 Inhale and stretch the leg.

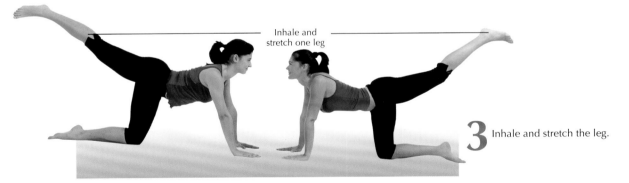

First three times with one leg and then with the other

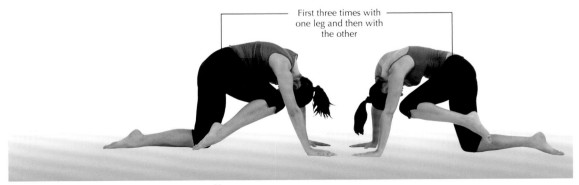

4 Bring your knees to your forehead.

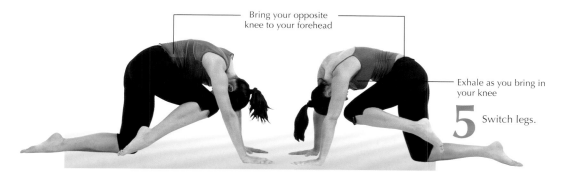

Bring your opposite knee to your forehead

Exhale as you bring in your knee

5 Switch legs.

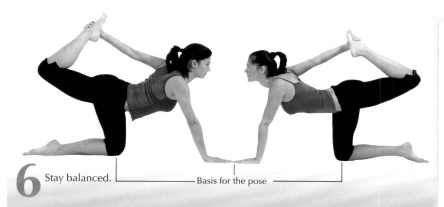

6 Stay balanced.

Basis for the pose

Benefits
- Mobilizes the entire spine.
- The vertebrae become limber.
- Reactivates blocked energies.
- Strengthens legs and shoulders.
- Tones the body.
- Tones the buttocks.
- Activates blood circulation in the legs.

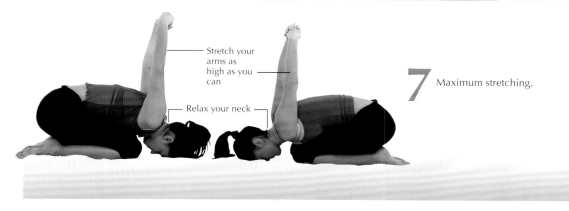

Stretch your arms as high as you can

Relax your neck

7 Maximum stretching.

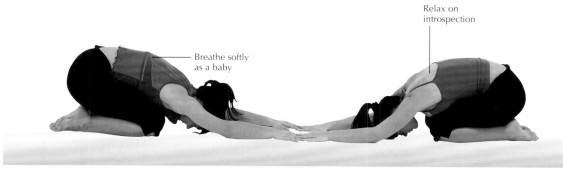

Relax on introspection

Breathe softly as a baby

8 Relaxation and rest.

Yogic principles
"First comes discipline; then joy"

1. Do not set any specific goals

Many people strive to have a flexible body, touch their knee with their forehead, or do a headstand (shirsasana), but this is simple competitiveness. These types of goals require that you use your mind, which seeks to "reach" a goal. Practicing any yoga pose has to be comfortable to the point of feeling pleasure.

2. Practice on a hard and flat surface

Asanas should not be practiced on slopes, near electronic devices, or on very soft, slippery, or rough surfaces.

3. Wear loose, comfortable clothing

When practicing yoga, wear natural materials like cotton, and avoid wearing wool, denim, or synthetic fibers. In the summertime, it is very pleasant to do asanas in a swimsuit or naked to feel air and prana on the skin.

4. Holding each asana

In the summertime, it is very pleasant to do asanas in a swimsuit or naked to feel air and prana on the skin.

Each position must be held for thirty seconds to five minutes, depending on the flexibility of your body (especially of the spine), your age, and your purpose. Asanas can be done in motion, especially for morning practice. When you hold each posture right, your body, breath, and mind will be in harmony and give you pleasure.

5. Principle of pose and counterpose

As a general rule, any backbend needs to be offset by two forward bends.

6. Caring for the spine as a treasure

For yoga, the spine is the "tree of life." Thus, people are either young or old depending on how flexible their cervical vertebrae are. The body's well-being depends on the condition of the entire spine. In addition, keep your back straight to allow kundalini to travel up to the top of the head to the seventh chakra.

7. Maintain discipline

A typical error of yoga practitioners is to give in to laziness. At first, most people are fascinated with the results, but then practicing gives way to work schedules, children, family obligations . . . and it is precisely then that more should be practiced! The only requirement for getting results is discipline, an obstacle that every yogi must overcome.

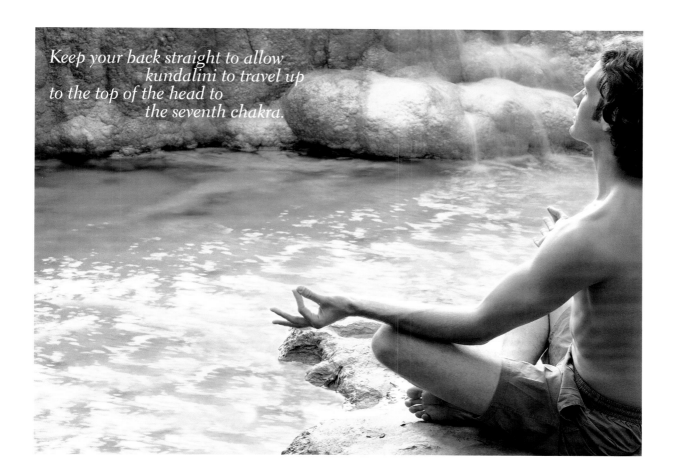

Keep your back straight to allow kundalini to travel up to the top of the head to the seventh chakra.

8. Personalize your classes

In this book you will find different ways of practicing yoga depending on your weight, occupation, fitness level, etc. For each individual there will be specific rhythm and poses.

9. Practice regularly

Set aside some time to practice yoga. The asanas can be done early in the morning (dynamic and moderate speed to awaken the body, since the predominant energy is yang or active) or in the afternoon (at a slower pace using various asanas for more muscle tone). Think of your practice as a sacred rite without interruptions for 45 minutes to an hour. If you do your asanas in the morning you will feel invigorated throughout the day, both physically and mentally. But if you do it in the evening or at night (when energy becomes yin or passive) you will be more relaxed and meditative.

10. Shower before each session

Never shower right after practicing yoga because water removes most of its benefits. Actually, only shower before practicing, as this will loosen up your muscles and enliven your mental state. Showering cleanses your aura or energy field.

If you do your asanas in the morning you will feel invigorated throughout the day.

11. Practice on an empty stomach

Wait at least two hours after your last meal. If you practice asanas on a full stomach, you will feel dizziness and nausea. Many advanced yogis practice asanas while fasting, which greatly increases their energy. Although I am not in favor of prolonged fasting, it is good to devote one day a week to cleansing the digestive system.

12. Do not obsess over results

Do not obsess over doing difficult asanas or increasing your flexibility by setting specific goals; it is better to let your practice surprise you. I remember one day I felt that it was time for me to try doing the chakrasana, the wheel pose with my hands and feet on the ground while arching my back and looking up at the sky.

It is a relatively difficult asana, but I already had experience. I felt it was time to try it, and sure enough I was able to do it. I was very happy with myself when I finished, but it was not self-imposed; there was something in me that let me do it, which is very different than competing with yourself or feeling restless about doing this or that position. I have also known people who say things like, "I used to be able to get into that pose long ago; could I do it now?" If you have not practiced in a while, do not assume that you will be able to do it as well as before, because surely your body will be stiff, cold, and will not have the same elasticity.

Do not compete with yourself and do not set strict goals.

13. Comfort, stillness, and permanence

These are three crucial aspects for doing asanas. First of all, you have to be comfortable in the position, and never feel pain or heavy tension in any part of the body (except for your back). Yoga sequences should be pleasant, so it is better if you are less flexible but more joyful. Time and persistence with every pose lets your body stretch more and be more relaxed.

New stimulating sutras

Let me elaborate new sutras to motivate yoga practitioners with enthusiasm so they can defeat their worst enemy: laziness.

1. Yoga is a smart, natural way of living in the world with joy and awareness.

2. The first purpose of practicing yoga is physical well-being, elevating energy, expressing emotions, understanding the mind, and spiritual enlightenment.

3. The benefits of yoga are immediate.

4. If you are attached to your routine, your computer, and laziness . . . jump before it is too late!

5. Yoga is aimed at those beginning to grow spiritually, and it is not a quick solution for existential problems.

Stillness is the basis for each pose; it is true that some sequences are more forceful but most require a long time for their effects to be felt in the body and mind. Hold each asana for the time indicated and come out of it gently.

And think of breathing as a silent binding code.

14. Breathe consciously

Every inhalation allows new energy to flow through the body's bioelectric current. And each exhalation is the expulsion of waste and toxins, as well as energy that got blocked by lack of movement or dormant emotions. Inhaling and exhaling through the nose is much more than we think: it provides important cellular oxygenation, awakens the brain and consciousness, and increases energy level to feed the chakras.

6. Practicing yoga prevents pain and disease. In fact, each yogi thinks of health as his natural state.

7. Youth is measured by how flexible your spine is, not by your date of birth.

8. Happiness is a common trait among yoga practitioners. Stay away from serious people.

9. Breathing is a bridge that activates your chakras and your emotions, and calms that "crazy monkey" inside your head.

10. Yoga will "burst" an inflated ego.

11. Do not think that because you practice yoga you are somehow superior; you are simply using your consciousness and your body's flexibility for personal development.

12. Do not resist the asanas . . . enjoy them!

13. Observe your mind as though you were on top of a mountain or an eagle in flight. Do not identify yourself with your thoughts; let them pass.

14. If you used to practice yoga before and you enjoyed it . . . why not continue? The benefits of yoga do not accumulate; you must practice it regularly.

15. Yoga is not just a series of physical poses; it is having a flexible, healthy, vibrant, celebratory, attentive, positive, and spiritual attitude.

16. A good yogi practices 24 hours a day.

17. If you think you have no time to practice asanas, pranayama, and meditation, do not worry. Meditate during work, love your partner consciously, look after your children with devotion, do business honestly, be creative in the kitchen and during your phone conversations, mind your posture while sitting at a computer, clean the windows of your house slowly and quietly, water your plants, sing when you awaken . . . that is also yoga, and it does not take extra time!

18. Eliminate every excuse.

19. Do not obsess over it.

20. Yoga will channel your sexual energy into creativity, economic success, spirituality, universal love, and your center. You will live in balance between what you feel and what you think, and have more clarity to satisfy your desires.

Sun Salutation
Surya namaskar

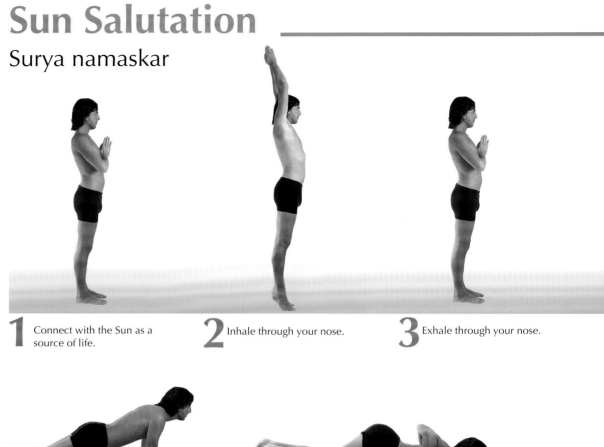

1 Connect with the Sun as a source of life.

2 Inhale through your nose.

3 Exhale through your nose.

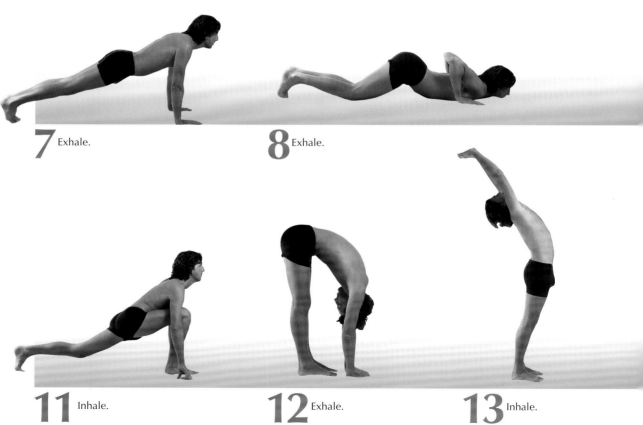

7 Exhale.

8 Exhale.

11 Inhale.

12 Exhale.

13 Inhale.

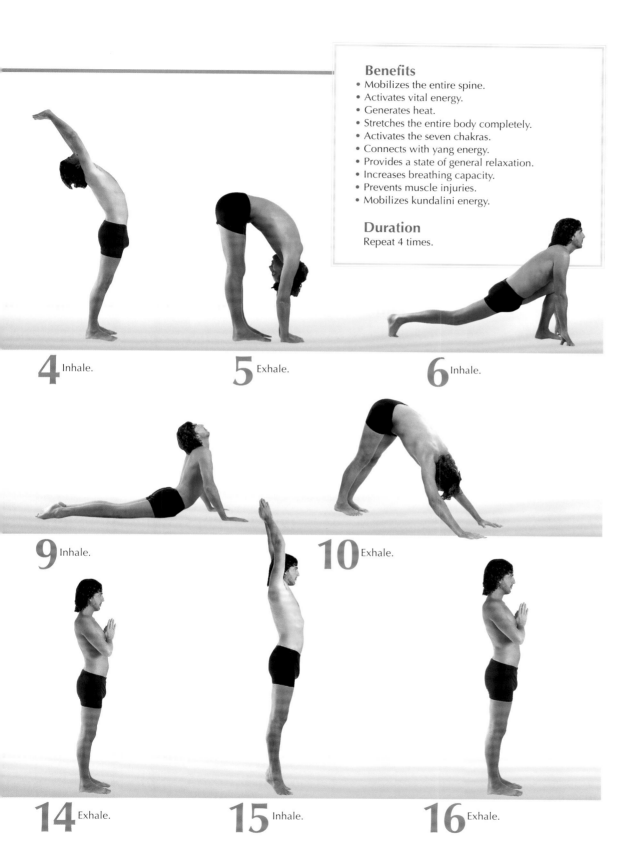

Benefits
- Mobilizes the entire spine.
- Activates vital energy.
- Generates heat.
- Stretches the entire body completely.
- Activates the seven chakras.
- Connects with yang energy.
- Provides a state of general relaxation.
- Increases breathing capacity.
- Prevents muscle injuries.
- Mobilizes kundalini energy.

Duration
Repeat 4 times.

4 Inhale.

5 Exhale.

6 Inhale.

9 Inhale.

10 Exhale.

14 Exhale.

15 Inhale.

16 Exhale.

Moon Salutation
Chandra namaskar

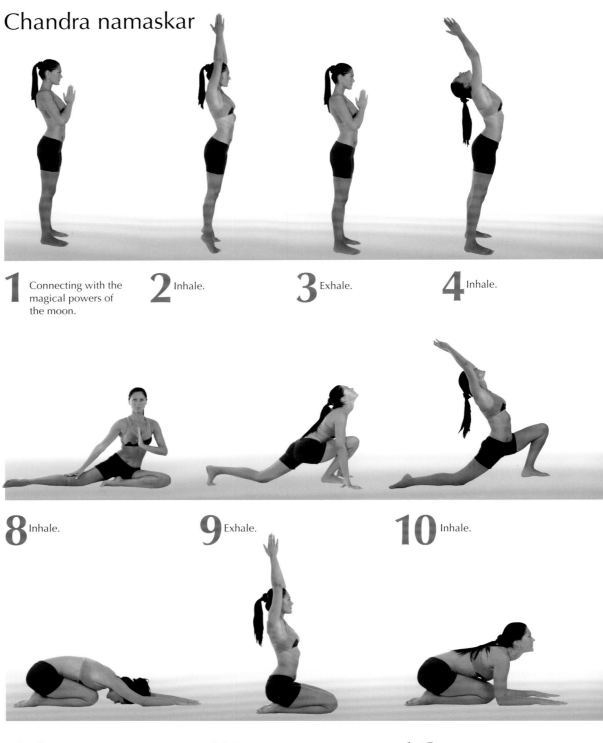

1 Connecting with the magical powers of the moon.

2 Inhale.

3 Exhale.

4 Inhale.

8 Inhale.

9 Exhale.

10 Inhale.

14 Exhale.

15 Inhale and exhale.

16 Inhale.

Benefits
- Connects to yin energy.
- Energizes the whole body.
- Activates kundalini.
- Mobilizes all areas of the body.

Duration
Repeat 4 times

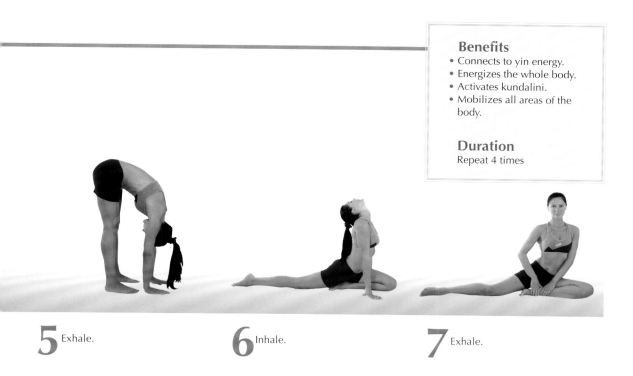

5 Exhale.   **6** Inhale.   **7** Exhale.

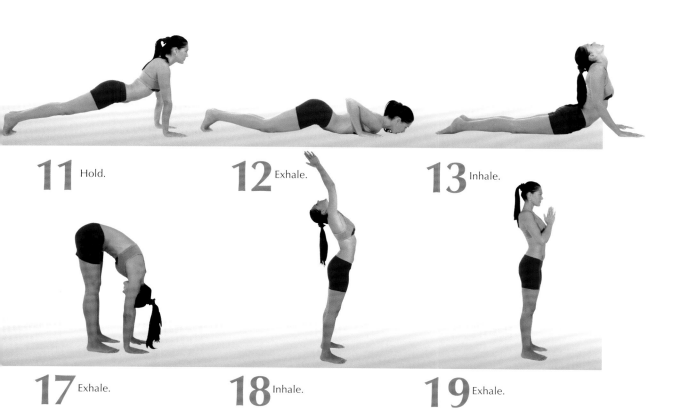

11 Hold.   **12** Exhale.   **13** Inhale.

17 Exhale.   **18** Inhale.   **19** Exhale.

Crane Salutation
Garuda Namaskar

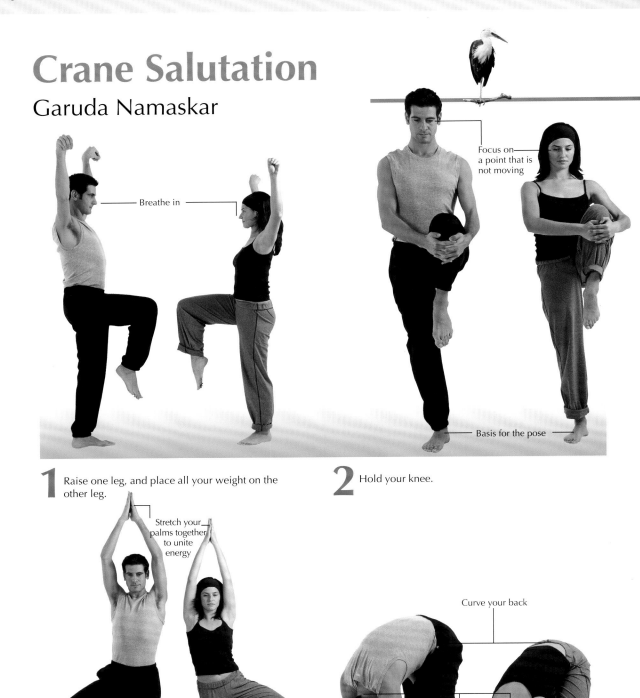

Breathe in

Focus on a point that is not moving

Basis for the pose

1 Raise one leg, and place all your weight on the other leg.

2 Hold your knee.

Stretch your palms together to unite energy

Stand firm

Curve your back

Relax your neck

5 Rest your foot on the inside of your other leg. Breathe deeply.

6 Using your arms, lower your head slowly and carefully.

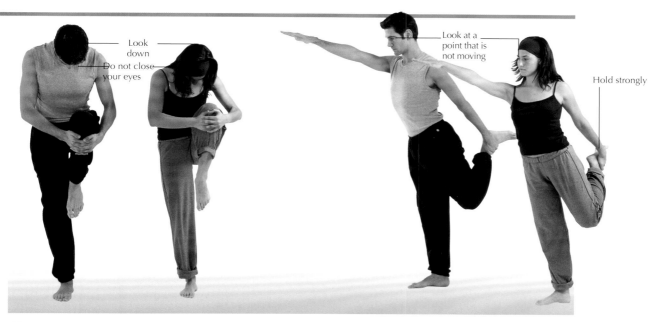

Look
down
Do not close
your eyes

Look at a
point that is
not moving

Hold strongly

3 Lower your head to stretch the vertebrae.

4 Work on your physical and emotional balance.

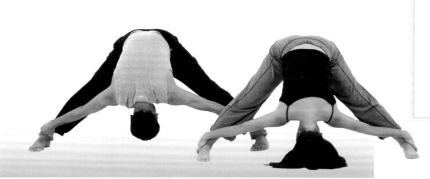

Benefits
- Provides physical balance.
- Stabilizes the mind and thoughts.
- Benefits the knee joints.
- Stretches both legs and back.
- Strengthens the ankles.
- Provides self-confidence.

7 Come up, open your legs, and grab your ankles with your hands.

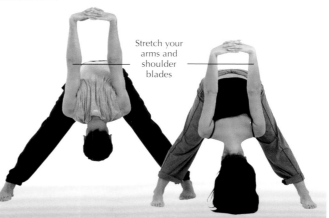

Stretch your
arms and
shoulder
blades

8 Repeat this cycle 3 or 4 times. It works as a warm-up before doing still asanas.

Yogic dance
"Conscious dancing brings you back to your human nature"

By dancing in my tantra and yoga courses, I look primarily to rid the body of tension and repression. This first release of the body is followed by the release of energy. Music, rhythm, and cleansing breath will make our emotions and mind loosen their grip over us. The enormous power, openness, and inner joy that are experienced in ethnic dances are like a gardener watering flowers. You feel ancestral, natural, and connected to life.

Heat and energy awakened by dance is great for your physical body, and they serve as the perfect warm-up exercise so you can correctly practice asanas.

Since yoga is supportive, just as we can be fluid and flexible like a river, dancing with meditative awareness can make a profound change in our internal state.

Stiffness equals death; therefore, flexibility and lightness that come from dancing are a shot of natural energy and a treat for the body and soul.

Many people feel transported to a different place when they dance, and there is an explanation for this: if you forget about schedules, routine, concerns, and constraints, what else is left? Your personal growth: your strength, joy, peace of mind, sensuality . . . .

Dancing brings you back to your natural state that you lost along the way; it tears down barriers created by the ego, and repays debt with affection.

Whenever you dance with drums or tribal music, feel how your chest opens with every breath, how your cells and organs dance in unison, how your blood flows, how your muscles warm up, and how your soul flows. Breathing is the fuel that ignites energy. Inhale through your nose and exhale through your mouth at all times and stay conscious and alert to how energy rises through the chakras.

Kundalini is also activated through dancing and serpentine fire spreads through channels and feeds each of your energy centers.

Dancing is a form of meditation, and keep in mind that it becomes even more powerful when you dance with a partner because you get to exchange your energy and balance your yin and yang.

Dance until your body feels like a flame.

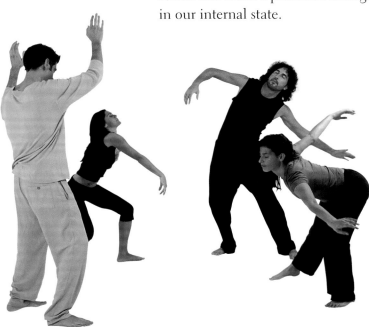

Ethnic dances

There is a variety of music and ethnic dances, but you can use your favorite music (I recommend drums and percussion combined with didgeridoo).

Breathe through your nose and exhale through the mouth, and give yourself permission to free different parts of your body as well as your spirit. But above all, unload your mind's "cargo."

Dance with your eyes closed, and if you suffer from "incessant thinking" (judging/thinking, competing, false shame, or another "virus" of the mind) wear a blindfold over your eyes to stop this mind chatter. Remember that you are not dancing for anyone in particular, but your inner being is dancing for the entire universe. It is a celebration, so remember something nice and celebrate it internally. Overcome every prejudice and dance as if you are half aboriginal and half a child, uniting consciousness and energy.

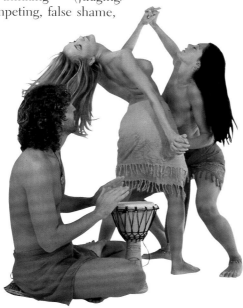

Dance is love
in motion.

In my classes, the participants have the opportunity to exchange partners and share each other's energy. There is a powerful enrichment whereby they become more aware of their energy and get in touch with the innate wisdom of the body and soul, not the mind. Dancing clears up any barriers created by bad habits or conditioning.

It opens up emotions, creates trust, and eases tensions. Your body gets unblocked, especially in the sexual area and the head, and you will experience joy, mental silence, and synchrony with the universe and all its Creation. In addition, it relieves back pain and releases emotional pain. Feeling a liberating catharsis is the biggest benefit of conscious, meditative, and tribal dancing.

Sequences for your upper body
Relieve stress, guilt, and tension in your neck and back

This series of poses is extremely useful for preventing pain and tightness in the trapezius, shoulders, and shoulder blades, as well as all types of cervical problems.

You should work on this area before each session to warm it up and remove any blocked mental energy known as "stress."

Kundalini energy fails to elevate if you are feeling physical tension. Contractures prevent nadis or meridians from distributing energy; they are like stones blocking a stream.

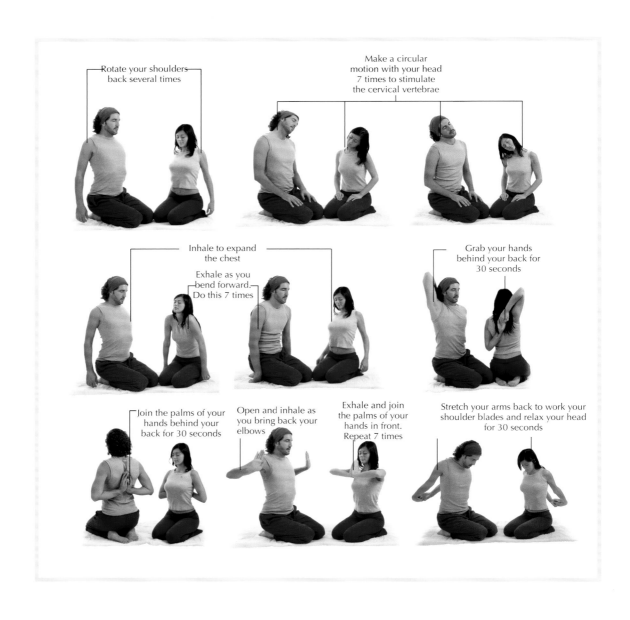

Rotate your shoulders back several times

Make a circular motion with your head 7 times to stimulate the cervical vertebrae

Inhale to expand the chest

Exhale as you bend forward. Do this 7 times

Grab your hands behind your back for 30 seconds

Join the palms of your hands behind your back for 30 seconds

Open and inhale as you bring back your elbows

Exhale and join the palms of your hands in front. Repeat 7 times

Stretch your arms back to work your shoulder blades and relax your head for 30 seconds

Pelvic movements

In the pelvis there is a huge flow of erotic sacred energy

This is an important movement to release stored energy in the pelvis, which results from poor posture, fears, guilt, shame, and repression. This phenomenon is more common in women, but today many of them are setting themselves free through belly dance, yoga, and meditation.

Do you know why the hip movement was repressed? Because any man can lose his head with the undulating, enchanting, magical, cosmic, sensual, provocative, and sexual movement of a woman's hips. And losing their head was equivalent to losing their power because male energy is in the upper body and feminine energy is in the fourth chakra, at the center of the chest.

The pelvis recycles and revives kundalini from the genitals to the brain, through movement of the hips, pelvis, and the first chakra.

Let bioenergy grab a hold of each one of your cells and experience the true power of the human spirit, as it opens your heart, spirituality, and sensuality.

One hand on the sacrum and the other on the pubis

Feet are firm on the ground

Exhale and inhale as you make a circular motion

Breathe through the mouth

Bend forward and backward vigorously

Focus on the sexual area and release that energy as you breathe out

Benefits
- Awakens the goddess within you.
- Activates sexual energy.
- Reinforces sensuality.
- Energizes every chakra, starting with the first.
- Eroticizes, releases, and spiritualizes your physical being.
- Liberates you from fear, low self-esteem, frigidity, premature ejaculation, and religious prejudices.

Duration
Each dynamic movement is done 7 times.

Balancing the hemispheres
Deep exercise to stimulate both hemispheres

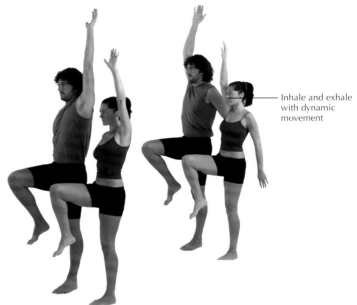

Benefits
- Activates the hemispheres.
- Warms up the body.
- Increases blood flow.
- Awakens energy.
- Strengthens leg and buttocks muscles.

Duration
Repeat for 2 to 5 minutes.

Inhale and exhale with dynamic movement

1 Raise an arm and the opposite leg at the same time. After a couple of minutes, switch to raising the same leg and the same arm.

2 Change after 20 seconds or so, again and again. This will create balance between the right side (yang) and the left (yin).

Union between heaven and earth
Movement in three phases

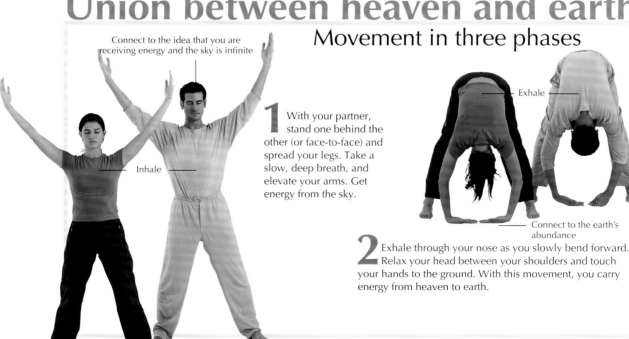

Connect to the idea that you are receiving energy and the sky is infinite

Inhale

1 With your partner, stand one behind the other (or face-to-face) and spread your legs. Take a slow, deep breath, and elevate your arms. Get energy from the sky.

Exhale

Connect to the earth's abundance

2 Exhale through your nose as you slowly bend forward. Relax your head between your shoulders and touch your hands to the ground. With this movement, you carry energy from heaven to earth.

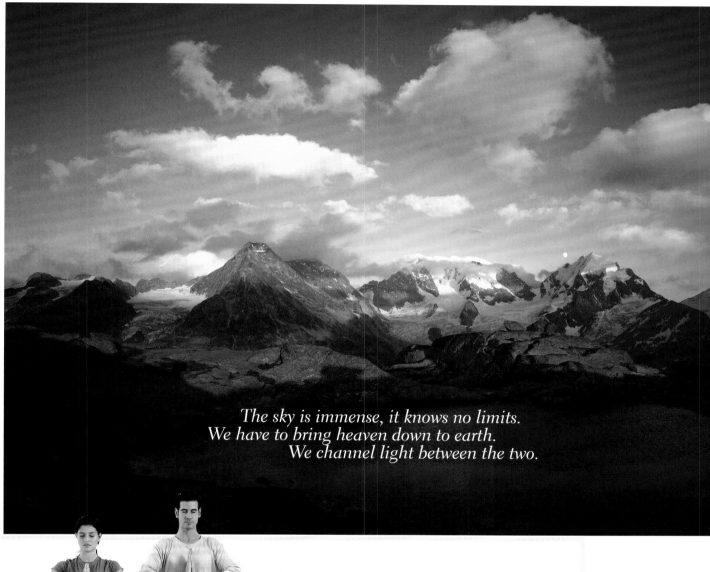

The sky is immense, it knows no limits.
We have to bring heaven down to earth.
We channel light between the two.

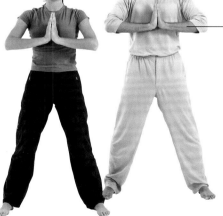

— Feel yin-yang currents together

3 Come back up slowly while inhaling and finish in pranava mudra by bringing your hands to your chest. Inhale again and repeat the process 3 to 10 times.

Benefits
- Absorbs prana and apana.
- Stretches the spine.
- Relaxes the vertebrae.
- Oxygenates the brain and heart.
- Eases leg fatigue.

Duration
12 to 25 cycles.

Open caterpillar pose
Greatly increased flexibility

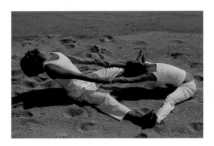

1 Sitting face-to-face with your legs spread, touch the soles of your feet and hold each other's hands.

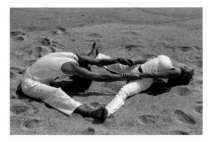

2 One of you bends forward as the other stretches.

Benefits
• Stretches your spine and lends more flexibility.

Duration
Two breaths each and then switch.
Do it for 3 or 4 minutes.

Caterpillar and fish
Warmth on your back indicates that there is an energy exchange

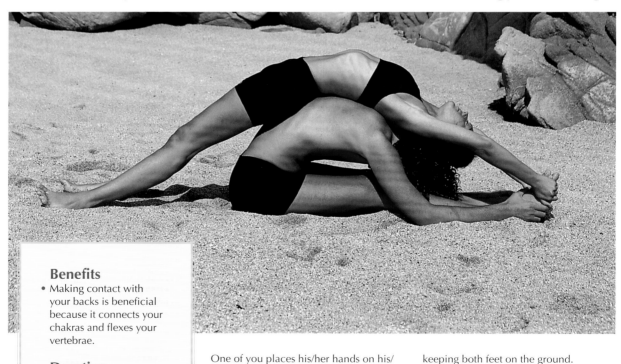

Benefits
• Making contact with your backs is beneficial because it connects your chakras and flexes your vertebrae.

Duration
At least 7 deep breaths.

One of you places his/her hands on his/her heels, keeping his/her legs straight while stretching his/her spine.
The other rests facing up on the partner's back until both necks touch, while keeping both feet on the ground.
Then switch positions.

Camel pose
Floodgates of energy open and fill with prana

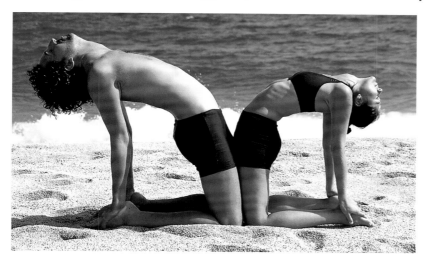

Bringing together your genital areas, hold each other's hips or reach for your own ankles.

Do a backbend to maximize the chest opening.

Benefits
• Opening of the solar plexus, heart, and throat chakras.
• Increased blood flow to the brain and neck decompression.

Duration
5 to 10 slow, deep breaths.

Upward bow pose
Containment and surrender, safety and flow. Yogic feelings of well-being

Benefits
• Decompresses and stretches the vertebrae.
• Completely relaxes the back.
• Provides assurance, support, and relaxation.

Duration
5 to 10 breaths.

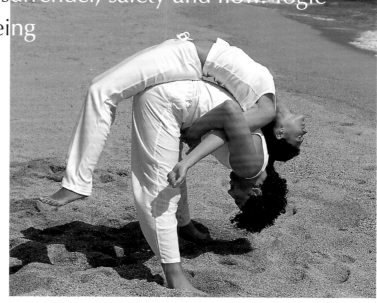

Stay still and place your hands by your heels, then relax your head and arms. Your partner climbs on your back, sliding up until his feet hang in the air. Lock arms with your partner and bend

your legs, supporting the weight of your partner provided that you both have similar weights. If your partner's weight is evenly distributed, you will not be straining to support him.

Finally, stretch your legs and breathe in unison.

Half-moon pose

Stretch to jump into mystery

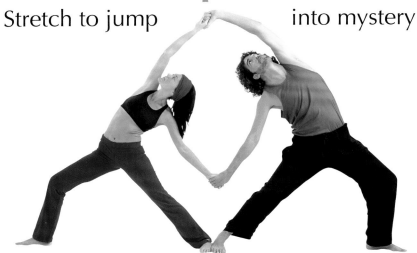

Benefits
- Opens and stimulates the higher chakras.
- Increases flexibility of the legs.

Duration
7 to 10 breaths.

Both of your right legs are flexed forward and the left leg is stretched far back.

Stretch your arms up above your head and try to reach your partner's hand, and

stretch your chest and spine as much as you can.

Full moon pose

Immaculate power of the queen of the night. Secrets come to light

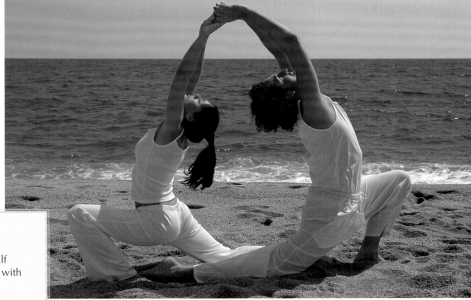

Benefits
- Similar to those of half moon, but stretching with greater intensity.

Duration
30 seconds to 1 minute.

Do a variation of half moon pose by flexing your front leg as far as you can; then, do the same with the back leg, so it is fully

stretched. In so doing you will form a moon in all its glory.

Child's pose
Share your inner sanctum with your beloved

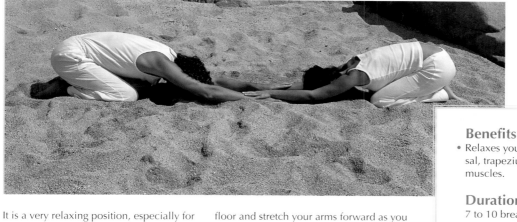

It is a very relaxing position, especially for the spine and neck.
Kneeling, place your forehead on the floor and stretch your arms forward as you press your hands down.

Benefits
• Relaxes your lumbar, dorsal, trapezius, and back muscles.

Duration
7 to 10 breaths.

Extended triangle pose
Vertebrae that are as flexible as the flight of an eagle

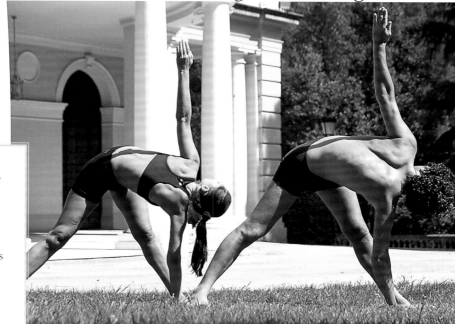

Benefits
• Rejuvenates the vertebrae by flexing its discs.
• Massages the digestive organs.
• Eliminates tension in the neck.
• Stretches your leg muscles and meridians.

Duration
Three inhalations and three exhalations as you lower your torso until completing three cycles on each side.

Stand with your feet apart and lower your torso, bringing your right hand to your left foot while twisting your head and looking at the opposite hand, which is stretched upward. Repeat with the opposite arm and foot.

Candle and bridge
Transmute your magical energy

Benefits
- Increases blood supply to the brain.
- Relaxes the heart.
- Rejuvenates all your organs.
- Eliminates leg fatigue.
- Activates the throat chakra.
- Relaxes all the muscles of the back, as you arch and flex your backbone.

Duration
7 to 12 complete breaths.

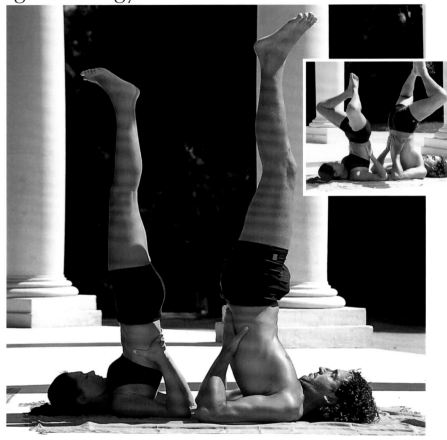

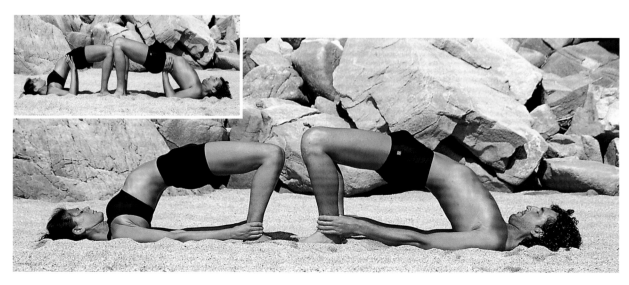

Do the inverted candle pose (sarvangasana) by supporting your weight on your arms, and avoiding tension at the cervical level.

Your partner does the bridge pose (setubandhasana), firmly resting his feet on the ground while lifting his hips. The head should be resting comfortably.

The arc can be done statically (leaning on the arms) or by moving the spine up and down. It all depends on your degree of flexibility.

Dancer's pose
Sharing the dance of the planets, trees, and waves

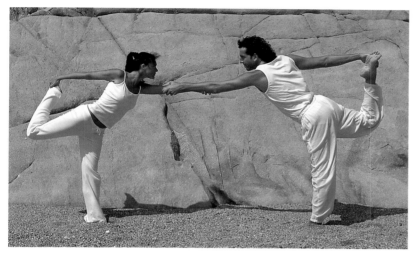

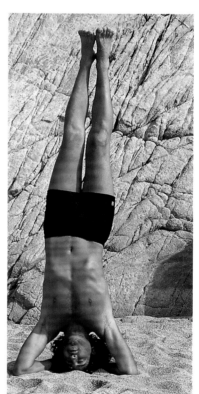

It is a balancing pose that helps circulate prana. Stand on one foot, grab your other foot with one hand, and lift up. Look at a fixed point for balance.

Benefits
- This pose gives you emotional balance through physical balance.

Duration
10 breaths.

Headstand
Become the master of your body

Benefits
- Brings blood and energy to the pineal, pituitary, and thyroid glands. Feeds the chakras with prana.
- Eliminates fatigue.
- It is useful for transmuting sexual energy into spiritual energy.
- Clears your mind.
- Increases endurance.
- Completely rejuvenates the skin and internal organs.

It is a source of youth and vitality because it goes against gravity.
- Benefits the eyes and vision.
- Stimulates the heart with increased blood flow.
- Helps digestion.
- Sedates the nervous system.

Duration
Start with 30 seconds until you get to 10 minutes.

*NOTE:
Inverted asanas are not to be done by those with hypertension, recent heart surgery, or brain or gland disorders.

This asana has the most benefits, but it should not be abused if you are just starting to practice yoga, and it is always better to have a partner to assist you.

The best way to learn is by doing it against the corner of a wall. Interlace your fingers, form a triangle with your arms, and support your head in your hands.

First, bend your knees and then push yourself up. Stay leaning against the wall, without placing too much pressure on the neck.

Tree pose

Balance your senses and emotions

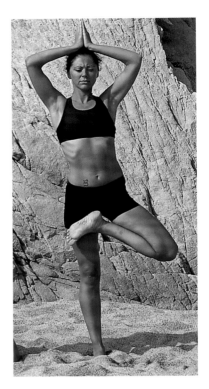

Benefits
- Develops physical balance and therefore, energy, emotional, and mental balance.
- Provides great serenity and trust in each other.
- Strengthens the legs, knees, and ankles.
- Increases concentration and calms the mind.

Duration
30 seconds to 3 minutes.

Standing on one leg, look at a fixed point.

Use your hands as a solid base for comfort and to get all the benefits out of this pose.

Shiva and Shakti

The universe moves through ebb and flow of the feminine and masculine

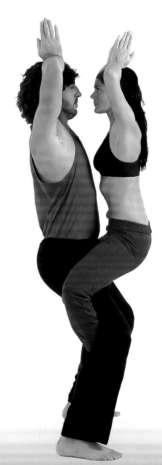

Benefits
- Connection in the seven chakras.
- Strengthens the legs and joints.
- Respiratory opening.
- Synchronizes energy.

Duration
30 seconds to 2 minutes.

The man stands, opens his legs, and bends them slightly to receive the yogini, who intertwines around him first with one leg and then the other. Then she uses her fingers to securely hold the asana at all times.

She will first lean on his shoulders, and then both will raise their hands over their heads, look into each other's eyes, and breathe in unison.

Pyramid pose
Ascend to the top of your soul

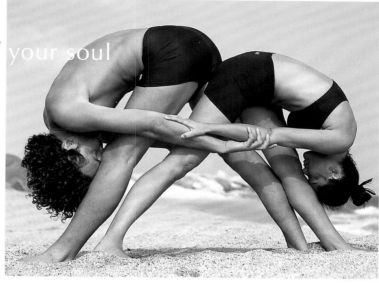

Benefits
- Strengthens legs and knees.
- Tones the buttocks and stretches your arms and shoulders.
- Stretches the vertebrae and corrects your posture.

Duration
1 to 3 minutes.

Stand on your feet, raise your hands above your head, and intertwine them with your partner's. Then slowly lower

until your legs are at right angles. It is very important to distribute the weight of the body to avoid a back injury.

Breathe in unison as you visualize the pyramid you are forming from the toes to the tip of your hands.

Bow pose
Shoot the arrow of your being to God

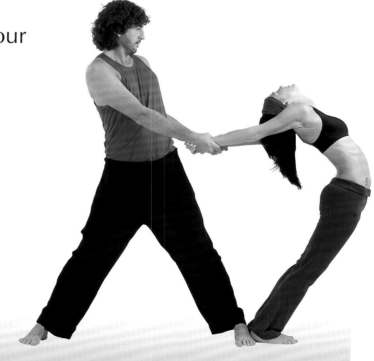

Benefits
- Arches your spine, thereby opening the solar, heart, and throat plexus. It is a pose for physical and emotional expansion.

Duration
20 seconds to 1 minute

Stand with your legs apart and grab your partner's hands. Your partner stands with his legs together.

He begins arching forward very gently, then exhales and bends back. And so, by forming a tense arc to

shoot an arrow and hit a target, the yogi prepares his body to hit the target of his soul.

Plow pose
Restores all your vitality

Benefits
- Eliminates leg fatigue.
- Increases body heat.
- Activates the three lower chakras.
- Massages the stomach.
- Stretches the vertebrae.
- Stimulates the thyroid.

Duration
10 to 25 breaths.

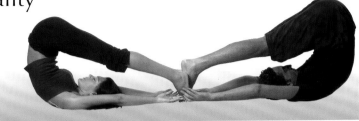

It is done in three phases: 1. Bring your knees to your forehead and use your hands to support your lower back. 2. Lift up your legs 45 degrees. 3. Slowly lower both legs and stretch them until they touch the ground. Then go down the same way but more slowly, resting one vertebra after another without ever looking up from the ground.

Downward facing dog pose
Climbing to the top of flexibility

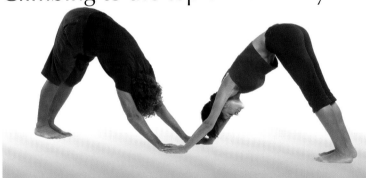

Benefits:
- Stretches the legs and arms.
- Strengthens the neck.
- Stretches the hips and stimulates the torso.

Duration:
30 seconds to 2 minutes.

Stand less than 3 feet (a meter) away from each other and open your legs slightly more than shoulder width apart. Take each other's hands under your legs. The back is suspended down, diagonally. Lift your head a little.

Benefits
- Strengthens the upper and lower back.
- Tones the buttocks and legs, increasing resistance.
- Develops self-control.

Duration
10 seconds to 1 minute.

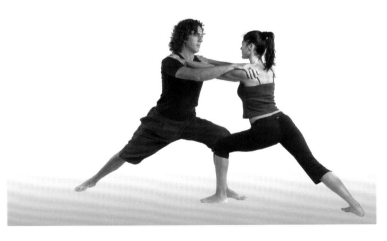

Stand at about 6 feet (two meters) away from each other, place all your weight on one leg and tilt gently forward with two purposes: grab each other's shoulders and stretch your back leg. This way your body will be straight. Look into each other's eyes.

Sacred encounter
Unburden your body

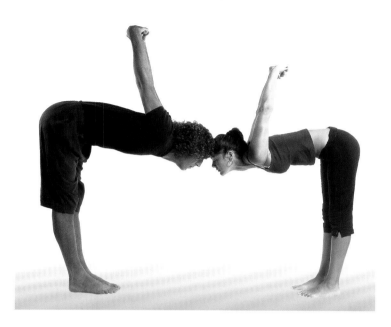

Benefits
- Stretches your arms and energy meridians.
- Releases leg tension by stretching.
- Connects you to inner centers.

Duration
1 to 3 minutes.

Stand 3 feet (a meter) away from each other and tilt to touch your foreheads. Your brow chakra (third eye) will open up.
Interlace your hands behind you as you exhale and bow down to touch.

Parallel caterpillar pose for your ankles
Connect with the earth

Benefits
- Stretches your legs and spine.
- Supplies blood to the heart and brain.
- Relaxes your neck.

Duration
30 seconds to 2 minutes.

Standing face-to-face, lower down to catch your partner's ankles, and then your partner does the same.
Make sure your arms, legs, and torso are fully stretched.

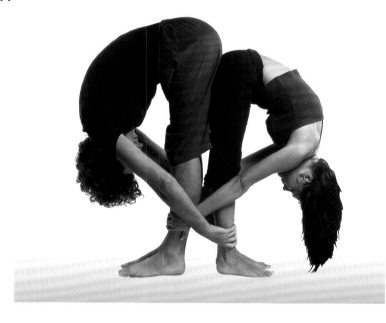

Yoga greeting

Namaste: your soul and my soul are one

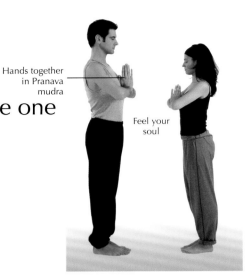

Hands together in Pranava mudra

Feel your soul

Benefits
- Increases awareness of the present moment.
- Prepares you for your practice.

Duration
15 seconds

Standing face-to-face, look into each other's eyes, and bring your hands together as a sign of devotion and salutation: Pranava mudra.

Extended Side Angle Pose

Stretch your sides

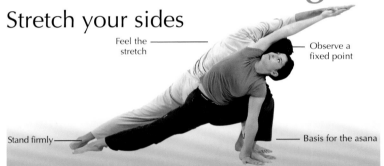

Feel the stretch

Observe a fixed point

Stand firmly

Basis for the asana

Place your back against your partner's, and bend one leg forward (left and then right) as you exhale.

Place one hand on the floor, next to your front foot, and flex your back leg as you reach with the other arm over your head and stretch your side.

Benefits
- Strengthens the legs. Fully stretches your sides and arms, increasing energy of the meridians.
- Strengthens joints of the knees and ankles.

Duration
10 to 20 seconds. Do it in a dynamic sequence—that is 5 seconds per side.

Dolphin pose

Bring fresh blood to your brain

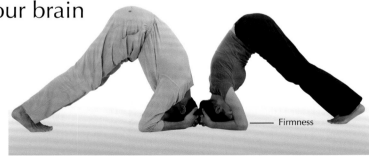

Firmness

Benefits
- Prepares you for inverted asanas. Supplies blood to the brain and tones the pineal and pituitary glands.

Duration
15 seconds to 3 minutes.

Bend your legs and then place your hands on top of the head forming a supportive triangle with the forearms.

Stretch your legs and stay on the tip of your toes.

Inversion with help
Receive energy from the feet

One partner supports while the other stands at a distance of about 18 inches (50 cm) away. The one holding stands with legs shoulder width apart, and the other grabs firmly with his hands, bends his legs, and does an inversion. The one standing grabs his partner's ankles and holds tight.

It is very important to keep the back straight and avoid sudden movements. Come back down slowly and stay in child's pose or cat pose for blood circulation to the head.

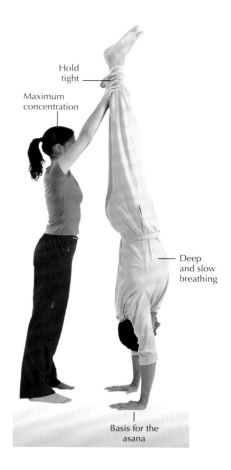

Hold tight

Maximum concentration

Deep and slow breathing

Basis for the asana

Benefits
- Increases blood supply to the brain and glands.
- Rejuvenates with an antigravity effect: energy enters through the feet.
- Tones the digestive organs.
- Benefits and relaxes the heart.
- Eliminates fatigue.
- Transmutes sexual kundalini energy by carrying it to the head.
- Relaxes and stretches the vertebrae.
- Activates all 7 chakras.
- Builds confidence.
- Sedates the nervous system.
- Increases breathing intensity.

Duration
10 seconds to 10 minutes. Begin slowly.

Contraindications
Do not do this exercise if you have hypertension, have had recent heart surgery, have hyperthyroidism, suffer from eye problems, or if you are menstruating.

Inversion with help (2)
Rest with confidence

This is a variant of the previous asana. Here, the one held supports her legs on her partner's shoulders (bends her arms and holds tightly) as he holds her by the pelvis.

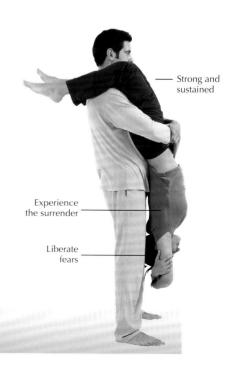

Strong and sustained

Experience the surrender

Liberate fears

Benefits, Duration Contraindications
- Same as the above

Surrender exercise
Surrender control

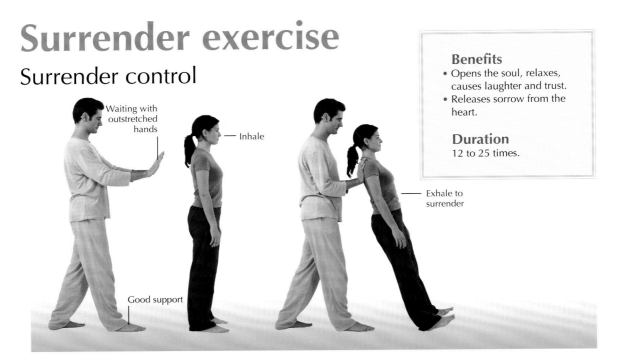

Waiting with outstretched hands

Inhale

Good support

Exhale to surrender

Standing with your back to your partner, bring your feet together and . . . let yourself fall back! At first you may feel fear, suspicion, and stiffness, but that is what was instilled in you.
You need to trust, surrender, and feel vulnerable. Like a flower, if you close up no one will know your fragrance; whereas if you decide to surrender to the dance of life you will blossom by trusting the divine.

Caterpillar pose with gripping
Prana flow

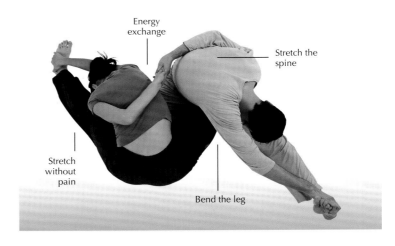

Energy exchange

Stretch the spine

Stretch without pain

Bend the leg

Benefits
• Stretches your legs.
• Relaxes the vertebrae.
• Improves shoulder joints.
• Massages the abdominal organs.

Duration
15 seconds to 1 minute.

Sit next to each other facing opposite directions. Bend one leg and place the sole of your foot on your partner's inner thigh, while stretching the other leg. Stretch the other arm and hold your ankle, and use your other hand to grab your partner's free hand behind your back.

Supine spinal twist
Rejuvenate your vertebrae

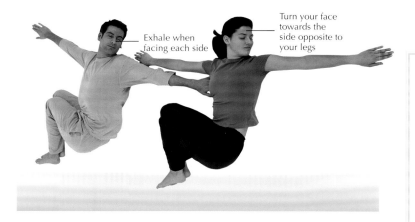

Exhale when facing each side

Turn your face towards the side opposite to your legs

Lying on the floor, bend your legs as your bring your knees and ankles together.
Stretch your arms out, turn your legs to one side, and face the opposite way; this produces an extraordinary twist on all the vertebrae.
Try to move according to your breathing; that is, inhale when you move to the center and exhale as you drop your legs to one side.

Benefits
• Rejuvenates the whole spine.
• Keeps your body flexible, vital, and light.
• Avoids back pain.
• Exerts an important stimulus in the stomach.
• Reduces your waist size.
• Connects your torso to your legs.
• Relieves neck pain.

Duration
10 to 15 times per side.

Double tent
Invert your point of view

Benefits
• Increases flexibility of the spine by lowering with additional weight.
• Supplies blood to the brain.
• Relaxes your neck.
• Stretches your legs and calves.

Duration
20 to 45 seconds.

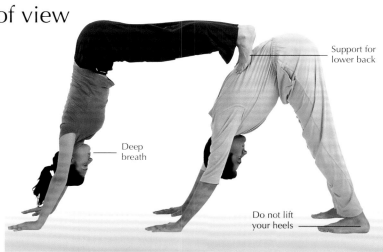

Support for lower back

Deep breath

Do not lift your heels

Standing with your legs open, bend down and touch the floor, stretching your arms. Your partner will place his/her hands on the floor and lift his/her legs on your back, placing his/her weight on your back area.

Five-pointed star pose
Five magic points

Standing back to back with your legs open, bring the palms of your hands together and form a five-pointed star.

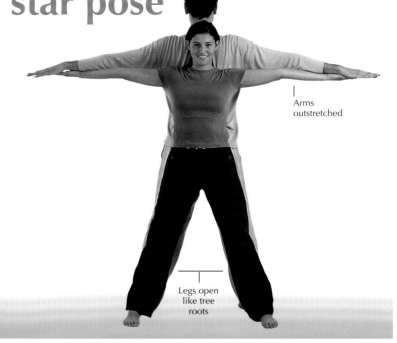

Arms outstretched

Legs open like tree roots

Benefits
- Exchanges energy and unity through the chakras.
- Increases your awareness of body heat and unity.

Duration
1 minute

Standing forward bend
Release fatigue

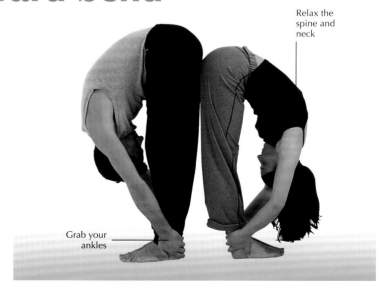

Relax the spine and neck

Grab your ankles

Benefits
- Increases vital energy.
- Recycles prana through the nadis or meridians.
- Increases blood supply.
- Improves flexibility of the spine and legs.

Duration
20 seconds to 1 minute

Rest your back against your partner's, stretch your legs, bend forward to touch the floor, and grab your ankles. Relax your neck and head.

Upward plank pose
Strengthen your body

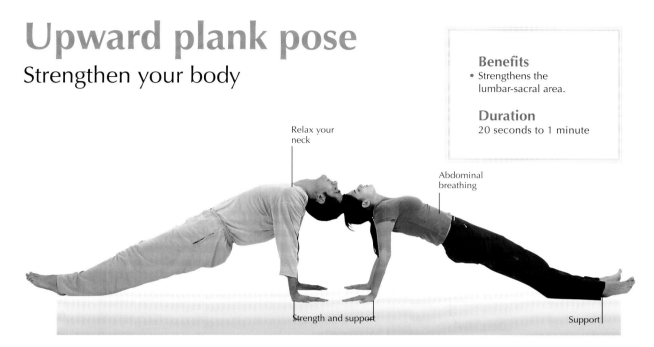

Relax your neck

Abdominal breathing

Strength and support

Support

Benefits
- Strengthens the lumbar-sacral area.

Duration
20 seconds to 1 minute

Sit with legs straight and hands firmly on the ground. Inhale as you lift your torso and buttocks, and support with your arms and heels.

Stimulating the spine with help
Increase your flexibility

Benefits
- Stretches the vertebrae.
- Produces an increase in gastric juice.
- Eases pain in the upper back.

Duration
25 seconds to 2 minutes. When done, rest in shavasana or relax while lying down.

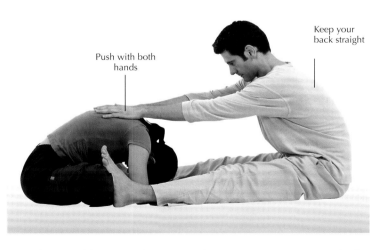

Push with both hands

Keep your back straight

Sit on the ground (bring your feet together or bend your knees) and lower your torso forward with the help of your partner, who will be sitting in front with legs outstretched.

These two asanas compensate for the stretching and bending of the legs. It is important to remember that your spine must not bounce, but rather it should keep still as you use your back to push forward.

Standing side bend
United like a rainbow of light

Benefits
- Warms up the back muscles.
- Increases flexibility of the arms.
- Reduces your waist size.

Duration
15 to 30 seconds.

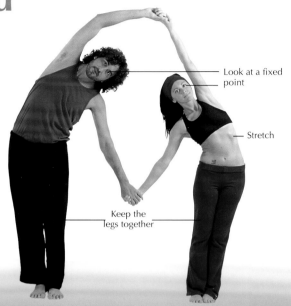

Look at a fixed point

Stretch

Keep the legs together

Stand with feet together, less than 3 feet (a meter) from each other. Stretch your torso sideways, then reach one arm above your head and keep the other arm down. Then hold hands.

Reverse warrior
Grow in every way

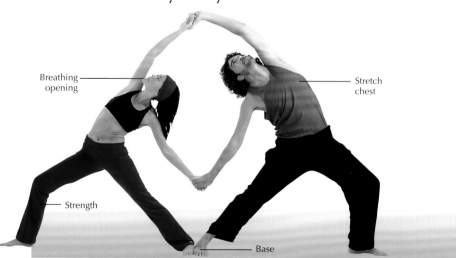

Breathing opening

Stretch chest

Strength

Base

Benefits
- Strengthens the legs.
- Opens the front chakras.
- Your arms and sides become more flexible.

Duration
10 to 25 seconds

This is a variant of the pose above; the difference is that you open up your legs, stretch one, and bend the other. Your feet will touch as you bend backwards slightly by twisting from the waist.
Finally, hold hands, as in the standing side bend pose.

Tree pose

They will know you by the fruit you bear

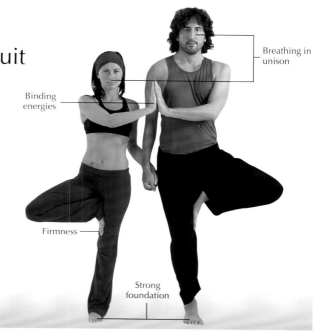

Breathing in unison

Binding energies

Firmness

Strong foundation

Benefits
- Provides physical and emotional balance.
- Activates the third eye.

Duration
1 to 4 minutes.

Standing next to each other, stretch one leg and bend the other so that your foot rests on your quadriceps.

Then hold hands and bring your other hand up to chest level. Gaze at a fixed point to stay balanced.

Warrior pose

Pillars of the same temple

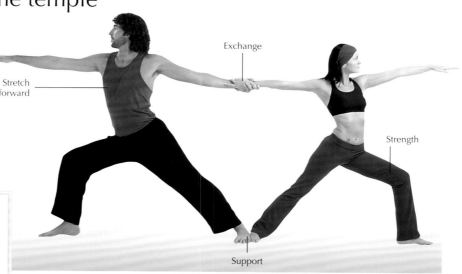

Exchange

Stretch forward

Strength

Support

Benefits
- Strengthens the legs, especially the quadriceps.

Duration
15 to 50 seconds.

Standing, hold your partner's hand while stretching one leg and bending the other leg forward.

Your foot meets your partner's foot for support.

Humble warrior pose
Order, consistency, and depth

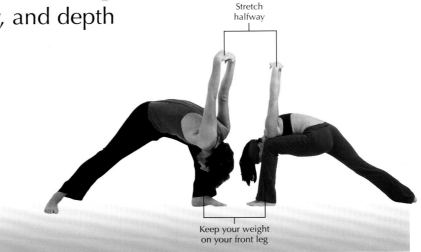

Stretch halfway

Keep your weight on your front leg

Benefits
- Gives strength and endurance throughout the body.
- Strengthens the heart.
- Stretches your arms and meridians.
- Increases resistance to fatigue.
- Supplies blood to the brain.

Duration
5 to 20 seconds.

Stand and bring your left leg forward and bend it as you stretch back your right leg. Stretch your arms above your head and relax your head toward the front leg.

Fish pose in a diamond
Open your inner doors

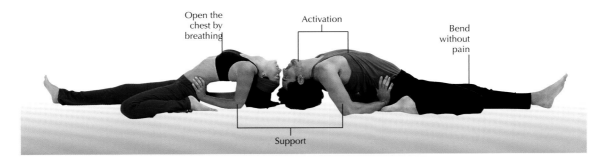

Open the chest by breathing

Activation

Bend without pain

Support

Sit facing opposite directions; stretch one leg and bend the other. Lower your back and head slowly, while supporting yourself on your forearms.

Benefits
- Opens the fourth and fifth chakra.
- Improves your breathing capacity.
- Stretches your leg muscles.
- Improves your knee joints.

Duration
25 seconds to 2 minutes.

Bow pose

Your body is a bow, your soul an arrow aimed at the divine

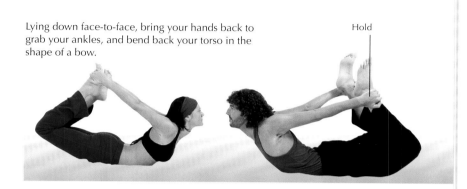

Lying down face-to-face, bring your hands back to grab your ankles, and bend back your torso in the shape of a bow.

Hold

Benefits
• Stretches and rejuvenates the vertebrae.
• Increases arm flexibility.

Duration
10 to 45 seconds.
You can also do it in harmony with the rhythm of your breathing: inhale up and exhale down.

Revolved head-to-knee pose

Side stretch

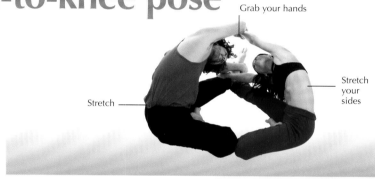

Grab your hands

Stretch your sides

Stretch

Benefits
• Straightens your back area, legs, joints, arms, and neck.

Duration
15 to 45 seconds.

Sitting face-to-face, bend your left leg inward and your partner will bend his

right leg inward. Stretch your other leg and reach your ankles while holding hands.

Head-to-knee pose

Love is not seeing eye to eye, but looking together in the same direction

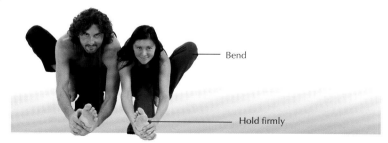

Bend

Hold firmly

Sitting on the floor next to each other, stretch your leg in front of you and bend the other leg so that your foot

rests on your thigh. Bend forward and hold your ankles with your hands.

Benefits
• Increases flexibility in the legs.
• Benefits the joints.
• Stretches your spine.

Duration
20 seconds to 1 minute.

The tigers
Journey from your natural instinct to cosmic consciousness

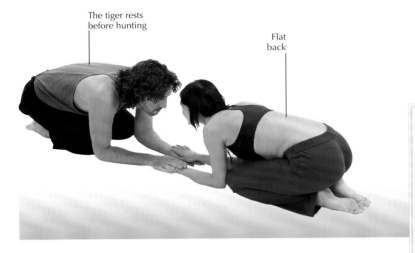

The tiger rests before hunting

Flat back

Kneel on the floor face-to-face, touch your buttocks to your ankles, and bend forward. Rest on your forearms, and place one hand over the other.

Benefits
- Improves leg joints.
- Improves digestion.
- Connects from the third eye.
- Relaxes the sacrum and spine.

Duration
1 to 3 minutes.

Lotus backbend pose
Open and rest

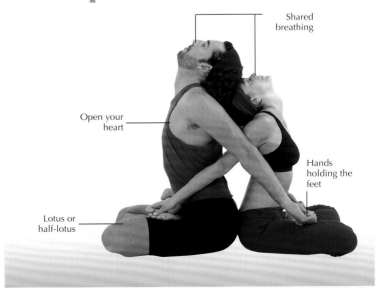

Shared breathing

Open your heart

Hands holding the feet

Lotus or half-lotus

Benefits
- Boosts energy.
- Connects all 7 chakras.
- Opens up the chest, especially the fourth and fifth chakra.
- Stretches your arms.
- Benefits cervical vertebrae and eliminates neck pain.

Duration
30 seconds to 1 minute and a half.

Sitting back to back, sit in full lotus or half lotus. Arch the spine and push your chest forward as you stretch your arms to catch your partner's feet.

Balancing lotus
Balance of power

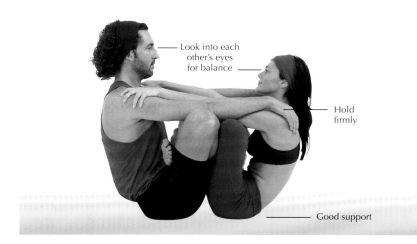

Look into each other's eyes for balance

Hold firmly

Good support

Benefits
- Opens the fourth and fifth chakra.
- Improves breathing capacity.
- Stretches your leg muscles.
- Improves knee joints.

Duration
30 seconds to 1 minute.

Sit on the floor face-to-face and sit in full lotus. Use your hands to lift your crossed legs.

Place your hands on your partner's shoulders and support each other. Gaze into the sixth chakra, between the eyebrows.

Yogic salutation in Lotus (1 and 2)
Honor your inner self

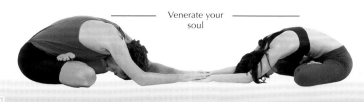

Venerate your soul

Grab the shoulders

Bend your legs

Benefits
- Provides greater internalization.
- Increases flexibility in the legs, arms, and spine.
- Improves stomach functions.
- Relaxes the head and neck.

Duration
1 to 3 minutes.

Sit in full lotus three feet (a meter) away from each other, bend forward, and grab your partner's hands (option 1) or shoulders (option 2).

You can then enjoy several minutes of relaxation in shavasana.

Magic chakra circle

Activate the chakras to expand the psyche and consciousness

This is an active and dynamic sequence to
share, unlock, and activate the energy of
the seven chakras.
Every move is related to a chakra, so it is
important to focus on the stimulated area.
Remember to breathe and feel.
Each full cycle can be done three times.

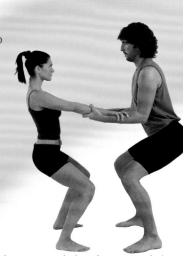
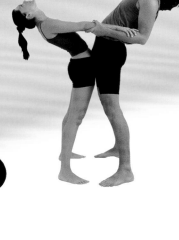

3rd Chakra

Stand with legs apart for good support, grab their forearms, inhale, and bend your
knees. When you go up (2nd phase), stretch your legs without letting go of the hands
and arch your spine and head back as you exhale.
Duration: 2 minutes.
Breathing: Inhale through the nose and exhale out the mouth.

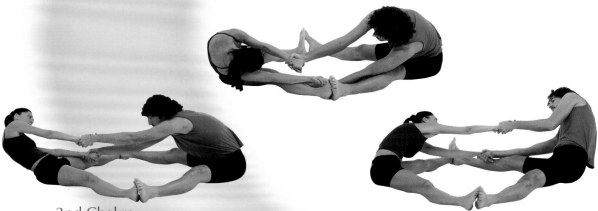

2nd Chakra

Sit with your legs open, facing each other; hold each other's hands and make a circular
motion from the base of the spine. (See the three phases).
Duration: 2 minutes.
Breathing: Through the nose.

1st Chakra

Squatting and holding hands, bounce up and down. Lift and lower
your genital area while holding hands. Look into each other's eyes and
breathe at a short, brisk pace.
Duration: 1 minute.
Breathing: Through the mouth, increasing the pace.

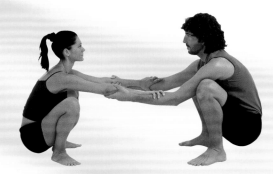

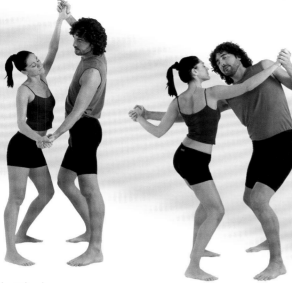

4th Chakra

Stand face-to-face and hold each other's hands. Connect from the center of the chest and dance in harmony and sweetness.
Duration: 2 minutes.
Breathing: Inhale through your nose and exhale through the mouth.

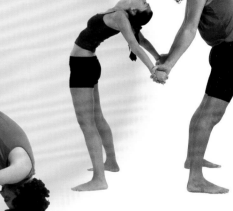

5th Chakra

With your backs against each other, join at the sacrum, bend forward, and relax the head. Stretch your arms back and grab your forearms. Inhale and exhale as you lift up your torso and say "Ahhhhhh . . ."
Duration: 2 minutes at a very slow pace.
Breathing: Inhale through your nose and exhale out your mouth.

6th Chakra

Standing face-to-face in the tree pose, stretch one leg, bend the other leg, and place your foot on your inner thigh. Raise your arms overhead, bring the palms of your hands together, and gaze between your partner's eyebrows, the third eye.
Duration: 2 minutes (if you fall, try again and again).
Breathing: Softly, through the nose.

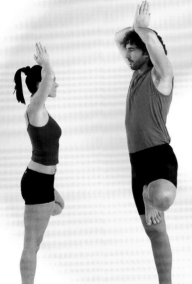

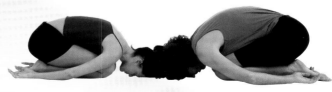

7th Chakra

In the child's pose, touch the crown of your heads and stretch your arms back.
Duration: 5 minutes.
Breathing: Through the nose.

Mantras and mudras
Activate the chakras using enchanting sounds and gestures

Sit up face-to-face in full lotus or half-lotus so that energy can flow directly between you and your partner. In the pictures you will see a different angle so you can better understand them.

This kriya potently stimulates the energy of the seven chakras through the bija mantras or "seed sounds" that correspond to their vibration, and mudras or gestures that subconsciously set off each person's inner potential.

The entire sequence is to be done in the same meditation pose, so do not stop until you have come to the seventh chakra. You can do a full cycle three times for each chakra. The first level affects the physical realm; the second, energy and emotions; and the third, your mental state.

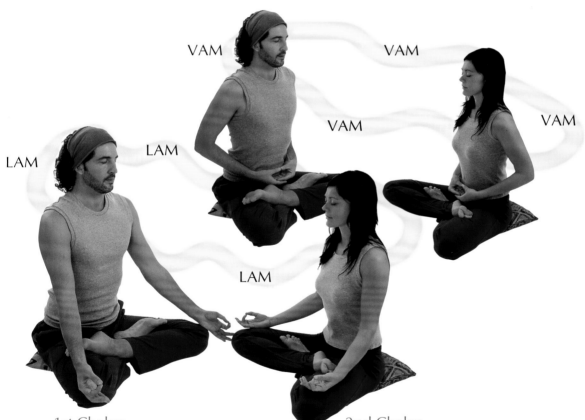

1st Chakra
Make a circle with your thumb and forefinger: Jnana mudra, or symbol of knowledge. Energy enters through the palms of your hands; it helps close an energy circuit and store prana within.
Mantra: LAM.
Repeat: Seven times for each one.

2nd Chakra
Shakti (woman) places her hands so that her right palm rests on her left palm and brings her thumbs to touch. In Shiva (man) the left palm faces up and is placed over the right.
Mantra: VAM.

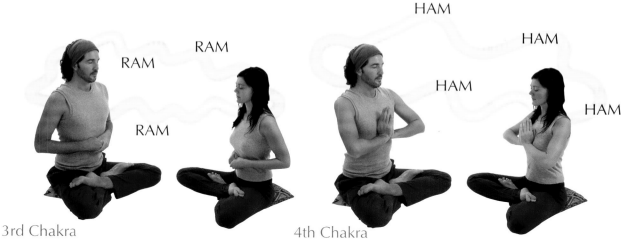

3rd Chakra
Touch the thumb and ring finger of the right hand together and close your fist. Use your left hand to grab the four fingers of the right hand and form a lock.
Mantra: RAM.

4th Chakra
Bring the palms of your hands to touch in the center of your chest in Pranava Mudra.
Mantra: HAM.

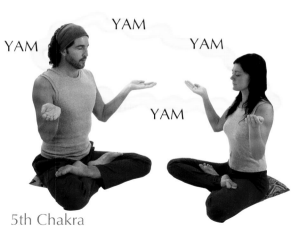

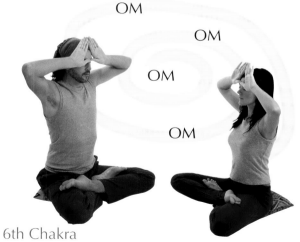

5th Chakra
Open the palms of your hands and lift them up to your throat. There should be no tension in the shoulders.
Mantra: YAM.

6th Chakra
Make a triangle with your thumbs and forefingers, and place it over your third eye. Then close your eyes and visualize that point.
Mantra: OM.

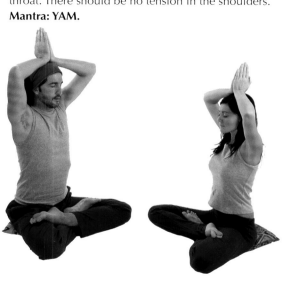

7th Chakra
Bring the palms of your hands together over your head.
Mantra: Silence, in order to feel all your energy flowing up.

Increasing balance and flexibility of the spinal column

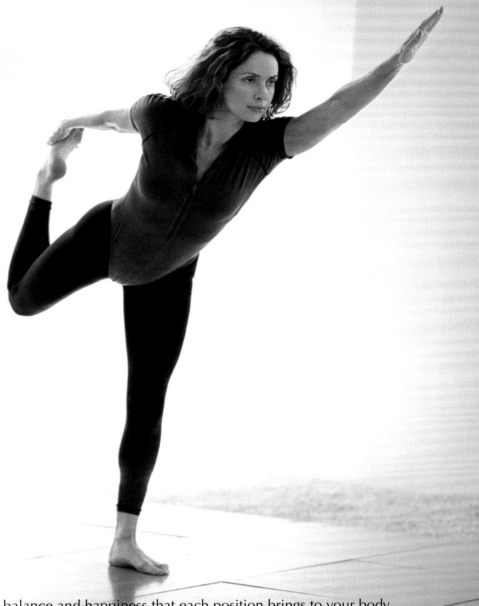

If you apply the balance and happiness that each position brings to your body and your relationships (partner, family, friendship), you will understand why yoga practice encompasses the body, mind, and spirit. You build your own temple as a great palace and yoga enriches your inner world.

The following illustrations will show you:

Dancing duo
The tower
Tantric temple
The gondola
Sustained flight
Half spinal twist pose
Tantric triangle
Locked lotus pose

Dancing duo

The spine is the tree of life

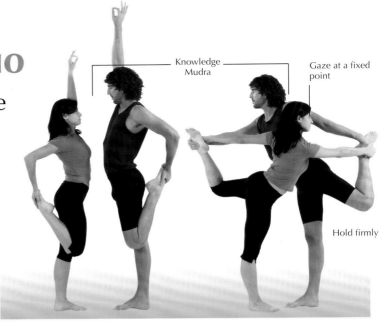

Knowledge Mudra

Gaze at a fixed point

Hold firmly

Benefits
- Increases balance.
- Brings energy to the third eye.
- Stretches the meridians of the arms and legs.
- Increases self-confidence.
- Energy exchange among yogis.

Duration
First phase: 10 breaths; second phase: 5 breaths.

Stand face-to-face about 19 inches (50 cm) apart, and bend one leg. Grab your toes with one hand and stretch up the other hand in Jnana mudra. Gaze into each other's eyes. This asana awakens intimacy, allowing you to come closer. Hold the position until you feel safe and then lean forward and grab your partner's foot. Focus on a fixed point for balance.

The tower

Look at the valley from the top of the mountain

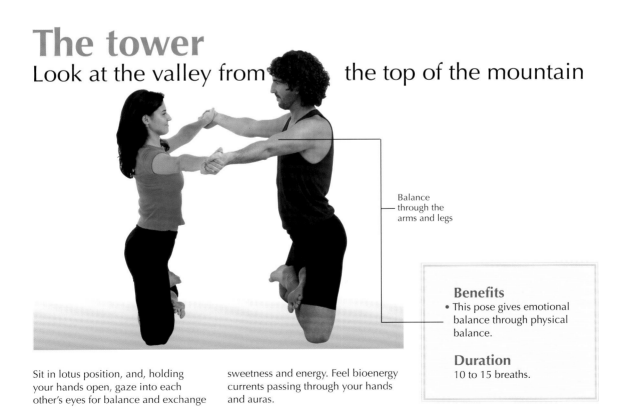

Balance through the arms and legs

Benefits
- This pose gives emotional balance through physical balance.

Duration
10 to 15 breaths.

Sit in lotus position, and, holding your hands open, gaze into each other's eyes for balance and exchange sweetness and energy. Feel bioenergy currents passing through your hands and auras.

Tantric temple
There is no greater temple than that of the human body

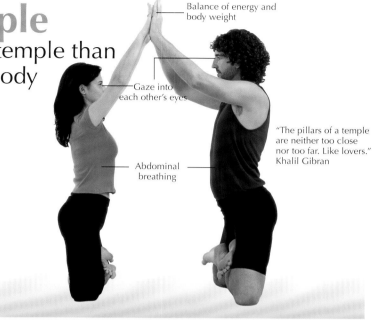

Balance of energy and body weight

Gaze into each other's eyes

"The pillars of a temple are neither too close nor too far. Like lovers."
Khalil Gibran

Abdominal breathing

Benefits
- Enhances unity among practitioners.
- Improves blood flow.
- Strengthens the nervous system.
- Increases emotional and energetic connection.

Duration
5 to 15 breaths.

It is a beautiful and powerful asana that creates a genuine energy pyramid: by sitting in full lotus your blood flow and energy flow moves up through the spine and it is distributed to the hands and eyes. Keep the same energy level and enjoy this balancing pose.

The gondola
Float with trust

Open the chest as you breathe

Relax your neck

Inhale

Hold firmly

Benefits
- Expands breathing capacity.
- Opens the fourth and fifth chakras.
- Improves flexibility in the vertebrae.
- Strengthens the pelvis and sacrum.
- Provides a sense of freedom and openness.

Duration
3 to 12 breaths.

One of you lies down on your belly, and your partner stands facing in the opposite direction. Stretch your arms behind you and hold each other's hands while gently arching your back until you feel a good stretch without pain or discomfort. Both of your heads should be relaxed.

Sustained flight

With greater freedom, there is greater unity

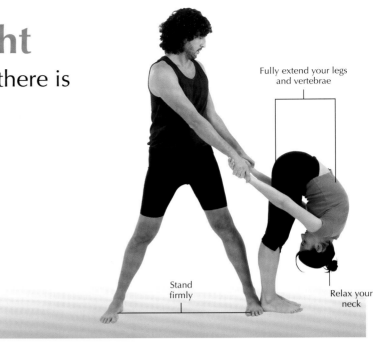

Fully extend your legs and vertebrae

Stand firmly

Relax your neck

Benefits
- Supplies blood to the brain and the thyroid, pineal, and pituitary glands.
- Stretches your legs completely, eliminating fatigue.
- Stretches your arms.
- Relaxes the cervical vertebrae.
- Activates the head chakras.

Duration
7 to 12 breaths.

Stand with your legs apart for good support, and your partner will bend forward while keeping her legs together and straight. Your partner will stretch back her arms to meet your hands, and relax her head as she stretches forward with each exhale.

Half spinal twist pose

Elasticity in the vertebrae

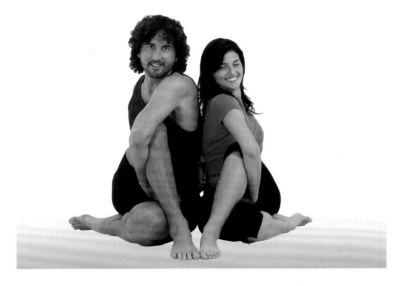

Benefits
- Revitalizes the vertebrae.
- Massages the stomach organs.
- Increases flexibility in the arms, shoulders, and joints.
- Repeat the same exercise, switching sides.

Duration
5 to 15 breaths per side.

Sit side-by-side, bend one leg forward and the other back, twist your torso to your front leg, and bring your elbow to the outside of your leg. Twist your torso slowly and place your other hand around your back to circulate energy.

Tantric triangle

Destroy the old, build something new, and sustain it with love and intelligence

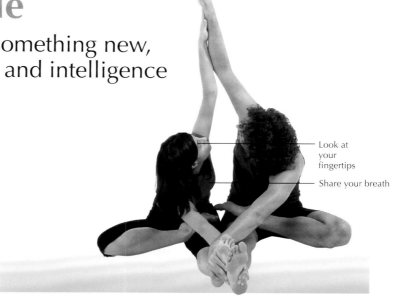

Look at your fingertips

Share your breath

Benefits
- Reinforces unity.
- Unites energy.
- Stretches your legs.
- Improves the knee joints.
- Strengthens the shoulders.

Duration
By sharing the sound and warmth of each breath you can extend it to 10 to 20 breaths per side. Breathe in unison aloud.

This asana represents the principles of tantric yoga: your hands stay grounded on your work and the world, but your gaze is directed towards the sky. The triangle represents love, energy, and consciousness—fundamental pillars for Tantra. Sit side-by-side, bend one leg, and stretch the other leg in front of you. Grab your partner's foot with your hand and reach your arm up over your head.

Locked lotus pose

Align the energy of each chakra

Sit with your back against your partner's in full lotus and lock arms. Inhale as you look to one side and exhale as you look to the other side.

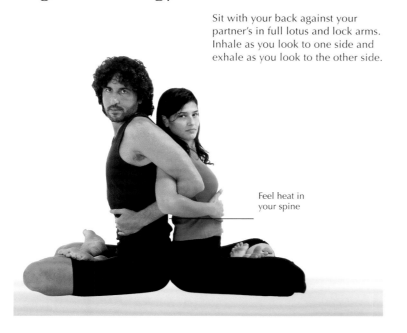

Feel heat in your spine

Benefits
- Unites the chakras and energy from the sexual to the spiritual.
- Provides a sense of unity by dissolving physical boundaries.
- As you turn your head you erase the past and the future, while remaining aware of the present moment.
- Generates strong heat throughout the spine, where your kundalini energy is shared after all you have done together.

Duration
10 to 20 full breaths. Do not forget to turn your head to inhale and exhale.

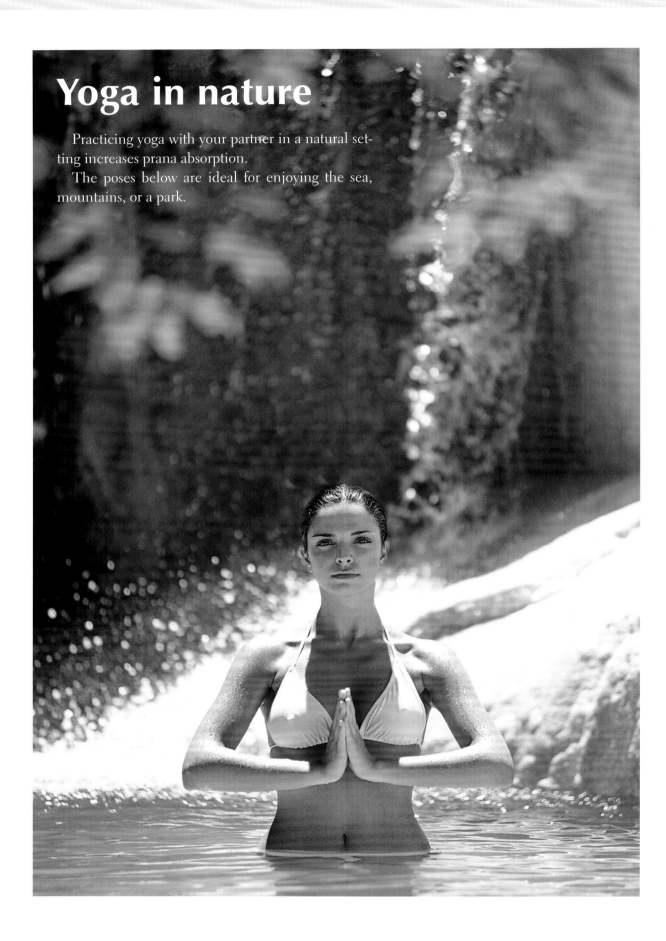

Yoga in nature

Practicing yoga with your partner in a natural setting increases prana absorption.

The poses below are ideal for enjoying the sea, mountains, or a park.

Warrior pose
Strength and expansion!

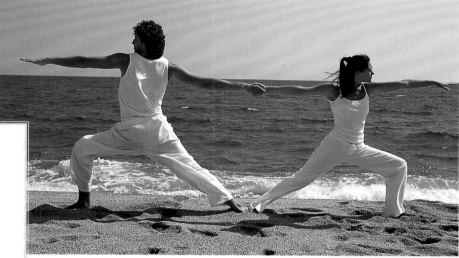

Benefits
- Strengthens and stretches the legs and arms.
- Balances your body weight.
- Strengthens the joints of the feet.

Duration
15 seconds to 1 minute.

Unlike the traditional warrior pose, here you each look to a different direction, feeling the yin and yang, right and wrong.

Supported shoulderstand
Irrigation and openness

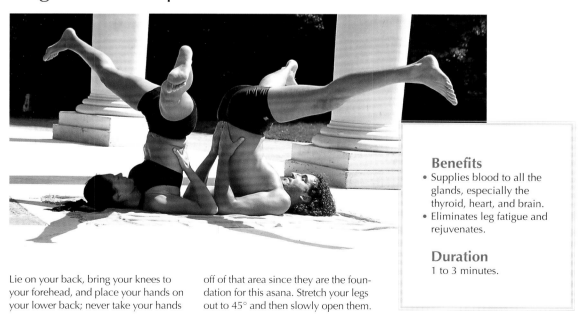

Benefits
- Supplies blood to all the glands, especially the thyroid, heart, and brain.
- Eliminates leg fatigue and rejuvenates.

Duration
1 to 3 minutes.

Lie on your back, bring your knees to your forehead, and place your hands on your lower back; never take your hands off of that area since they are the foundation for this asana. Stretch your legs out to 45° and then slowly open them.

Hip-opening seated pose
Share your sacred spine

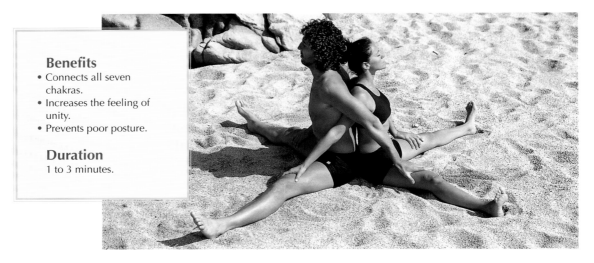

Benefits
- Connects all seven chakras.
- Increases the feeling of unity.
- Prevents poor posture.

Duration
1 to 3 minutes.

Sit with your back against your partner's, open your legs, and stretch your arms behind you to touch your partner's thighs. Keep your back straight at all times.

Bridge pose
Release tension from your lower body

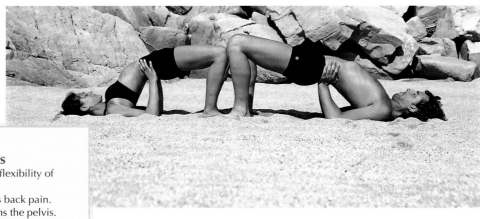

Benefits
- Increases flexibility of the spine.
- Eliminates back pain.
- Strengthens the pelvis.
- Activates chakras from the first to the fifth.

Duration
1 to 2 minutes.

Lying on the ground, open your legs shoulder width apart. Bend them so that the soles of the feet are flat on the floor, and bring your heels close to your buttocks. Then lift your pelvis as you inhale and grab each of your ankles. Hold the pose or lift up and lower as you inhale and exhale. For the second option, place your elbows on the floor for support and place your hands on the sacrum.

Chair pose
Power and strength

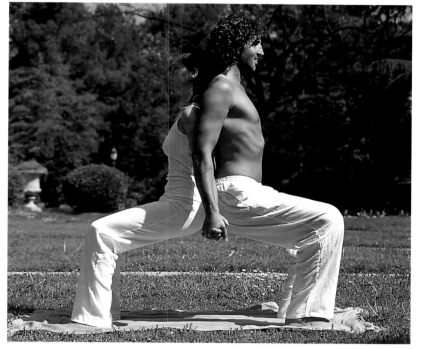

Benefits
- It may be the asana that most strengthens the legs, by supporting the weight of the moving body.
- It is also beneficial for the heart.

Duration
10 to 15 repetitions.

Stand with your back against your partner's, open your legs, and hold hands. In this position, inhale as you move your torso up and exhale as you come back down.

Fish and diamond pose
Open up your self-expression, love, and creativity

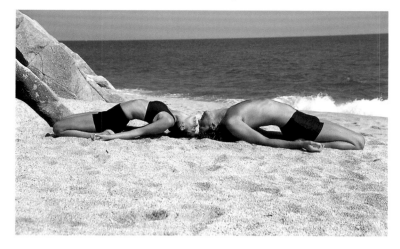

Benefits
- Opens the fourth chakra.
- Activates creativity.
- Deepens breathing, providing feeling of spaciousness and freedom.
- Prevents problems in the knee joints.
- Stretches your quadriceps.
- Supplies blood to the brain and pineal and pituitary glands.

Duration
30 seconds to 1 minute and a half.

Facing opposite directions, sit less than 3 feet (a meter) away, in diamond pose, on your heels with your legs bent. Then lower back slowly using your hands.

Bring the top of the head to the ground and push up with your elbows to hold the pose.

Frog pose
Become small and then expand

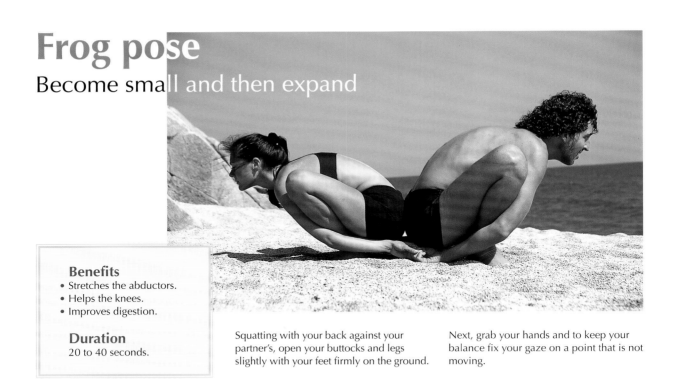

Benefits
- Stretches the abductors.
- Helps the knees.
- Improves digestion.

Duration
20 to 40 seconds.

Squatting with your back against your partner's, open your buttocks and legs slightly with your feet firmly on the ground.

Next, grab your hands and to keep your balance fix your gaze on a point that is not moving.

Head-to-knee forward bend
Sharing pleasure, relaxation, and stretching

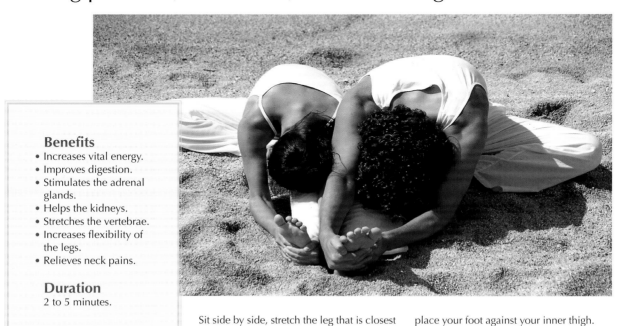

Benefits
- Increases vital energy.
- Improves digestion.
- Stimulates the adrenal glands.
- Helps the kidneys.
- Stretches the vertebrae.
- Increases flexibility of the legs.
- Relieves neck pains.

Duration
2 to 5 minutes.

Sit side by side, stretch the leg that is closest to your partner, bend the other leg, and place your foot against your inner thigh. Bend forward and grab your ankles.

Boat pose
We cannot change the wind, but we can adjust the sails

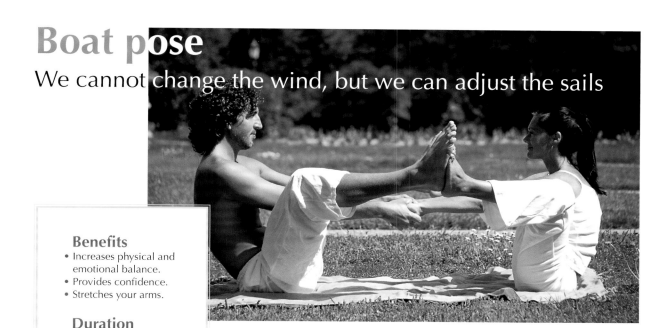

Benefits
- Increases physical and emotional balance.
- Provides confidence.
- Stretches your arms.

Duration
1 to 2 minutes.

Sit face-to-face, bend your legs, and lift up the soles of your feet. Stretch your arms between your legs and hold hands. Gaze into your partner's eyes and eyebrows.

Preparing for caterpillar pose
Increase your flexibility

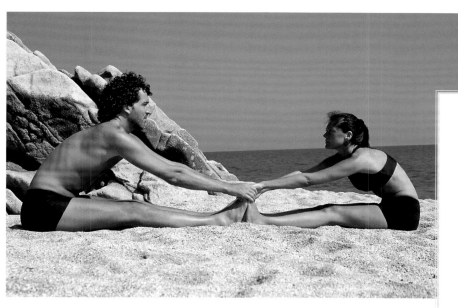

Benefits
- Supplies fresh blood to all the glands.
- Stretches your legs and the meridians, increasing the flow of prana.
- Eliminates fatigue.
- Stretches your arms and upper back.

Duration
1 to 2 minutes.

Sit face-to-face, stretch your legs as far as you can, and bring your feet together. Stretch your hands as you bend forward.

Wide-angle seated forward bend
Movement and flexibility

Benefits
- Provides great elasticity to the whole area of the spine and sacrum.
- Stretches and relaxes the entire leg.
- Generally gives you more flexibility with stimulation from your partner's weight.

Duration
20 to 30 times.

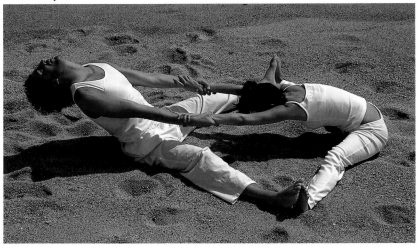

Sit on the ground, open your legs completely, and bring together the soles of the feet as you hold each other's arms or hands (not the wrists). Exhale as you bend forward and inhale as you bend back.

Child's pose
Venerate your partner

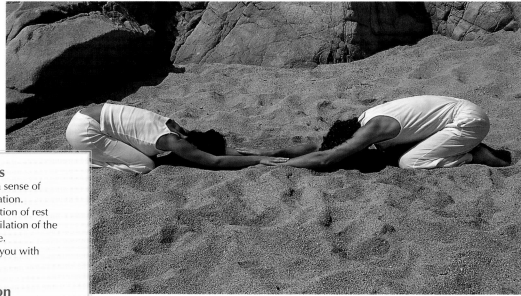

Benefits
- Provides a sense of internalization.
- It is a position of rest and assimilation of the work done.
- Connects you with Earth.

Duration
2 to 5 minutes.

Bend your legs and sit on your heels; bend forward. Place your forehead and hands on the floor.

Full boat pose
Navigate in the sea of emotional and physical balance

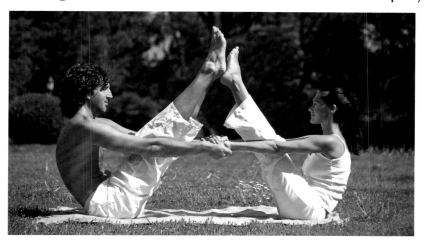

Sit face-to-face about 3 feet (one meter) apart, bend your legs, and touch the soles of your feet. Hold each other's hands for balance, and lift up your legs slowly until they are fully stretched. If you start to laugh do not hold it in, but bring back your focus to your body.

Benefits
- Stretches your legs deeply, eliminating fatigue.
- Develops a broad sense of balance.
- Gives you emotional and mental balance.

Duration
30 seconds to 1 minute, then undo and repeat 3 times.

Spinal twist in lotus
Rejuvenate your vertebrae

Benefits
- Deep stretch.
- Allows the vertebrae to rejuvenate as you move sideways.
- Massages digestive organs and viscera.

Duration
Hold it for 20 to 30 seconds, then switch sides. Repeat 3 times.

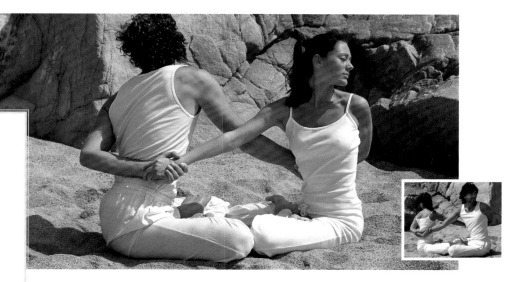

Sit face-to-face with crossed legs and your back straight, and twist to one side as your partner twists to the other side. In this position, hold each other firmly by the forearms.

Wheel pose

Spin your whole life, your chakras, and your energy

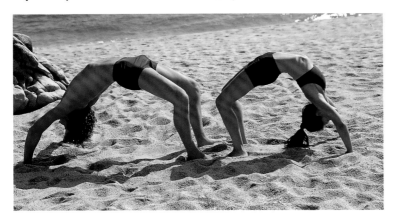

This asana will come with practice, and it is very helpful to have a partner to provide assistance. It can also be done on your own.

First, stand firmly on your legs with your feet shoulder width apart or a little more. Take a deep breath and stretch your arms above your head, do a backbend, and place your hands on the floor.

Gradually, using the strength of your legs and arms, build momentum and lift your torso until you form a semicircle. Your head should be relaxed.

Benefits
- Stimulates all the glands of the endocrine system and organs: gonads, adrenals, kidneys, spleen, thymus, thyroid, parathyroid, pineal, and pituitary. Enables its functioning completely to stimulate your psyche.
- Rejuvenates the movement of the vertebrae.
- Expands your breathing capacity.
- Strengthens your arms and legs.

Duration
15 seconds to 1 minute.

Stacked child's pose

Be a seed of light

Benefits
- Stimulates all your glands
- Completely relaxes the back.
- Promotes introspection.
- Increases flexibility of the spine by using your partner's weight as a stimulus.

Duration
1 to 2 minutes.

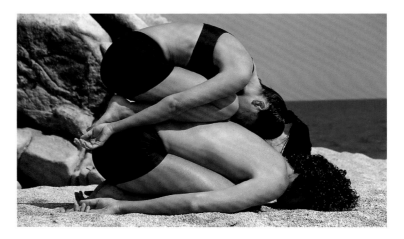

Kneel, bring your forehead to the floor, stretch back your arms, and relax your back, legs, and neck.

Your partner will climb on top and you will both look like twins. And to think, we held this asana for nine months!

Cobra pose
Stimulate your kundalini

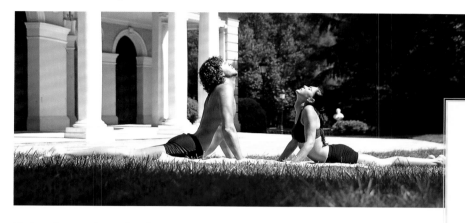

Lie face down with your hands to your sides, lift your torso, and tilt your head back. Push up with your arms, not your back, to avoid injury.

Benefits
- Activates the kundalini.
- Expands breathing.
- Stretches the spine and abdominal muscles.
- Strengthens the arms.

Duration
1 to 2 minutes.

Corpse pose
Yoga nidra: travel the inner world

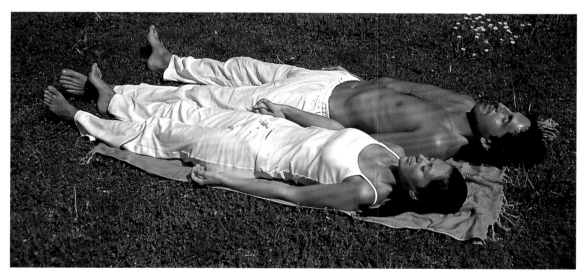

Lie on your back, relax your body from head to toe, and try to feel completely ethereal and light. Be more energy and less matter. Many practitioners live an out of body experience or "astral travel" because their body experiences strong receptivity to new energy which then circulates the chakras through consciousness. Do not be afraid and do not cling to your physical body; let it happen and flow.
At this point, relax and enjoy the experience. Your mind is silent and your awareness expands without limits . . . .

Awakening female sensuality

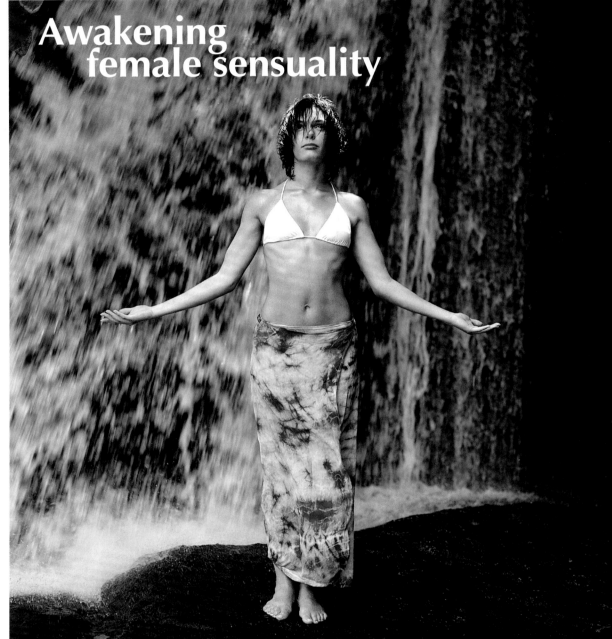

This sequence made between Shaktis enables women to practice yoga poses together and exchange energy and physical and spiritual unity with each other. Feminine energy, or yin, is receptive, sensual, erotic, circular, and we are now in the era when planetary Shakti is awakened, allowing the blossoming of the divine in its feminine polarity. And it is not by chance that the feminine is now being worshipped, at the same time that many women experience new emotional and effective relationships with other women; something that goes back to ancient times when Indian wisewomen taught the young ones the secrets of love, dance, seduction, and eroticism.

* These asanas can be done with partners of the opposite sex.

Tree pose

We are seeds of light striving to grow as a tree that bears fruits of love

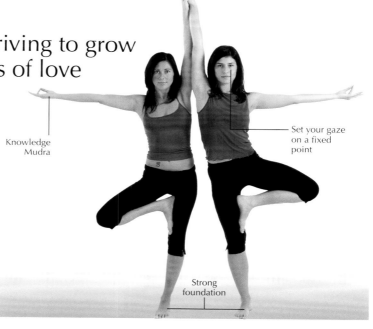

Knowledge Mudra

Set your gaze on a fixed point

Strong foundation

Benefits
- Improves your balance.
- Promotes concentration.

Duration
10 to 18 breaths per side.

Stand next to each other, facing the same direction; bend one leg and place your foot on your adductor muscle. Hold hands and stretch your other arm down. Gaze at a fixed point for balance.

Suspension bridge

Life is a river and love is the bridge that crosses it on the banks of the divine

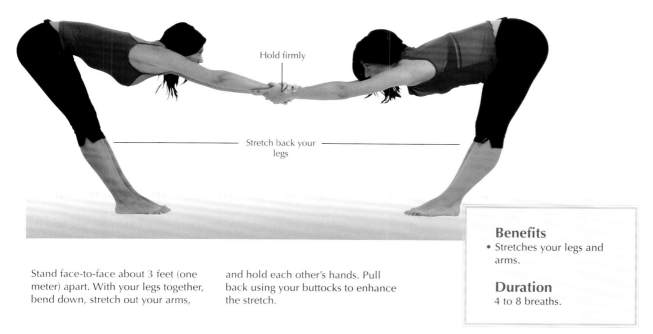

Hold firmly

Stretch back your legs

Stand face-to-face about 3 feet (one meter) apart. With your legs together, bend down, stretch out your arms, and hold each other's hands. Pull back using your buttocks to enhance the stretch.

Benefits
- Stretches your legs and arms.

Duration
4 to 8 breaths.

Standing forward fold pose
Stretch your legs to eliminate fatigue

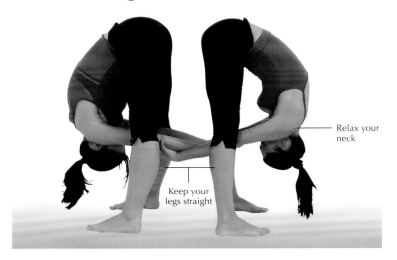

Benefits
- Strengthens unity.
- Supplies blood to the legs and prevents varicose veins and muscle spasms (so it is ideal for athletes).
- Increases youthfulness in the vertebrae.
- Relaxes your neck.
- Supplies blood to the brain.
- Activates the sexual chakra.

Duration
4 to 8 breaths.

Relax your neck

Keep your legs straight

Standing facing opposite directions with your legs shoulder width apart, bend forward. Stretch your arms between your legs and hold hands or forearms.

Standing forward bend with raised arms
When you stretch, your body rejuvenates

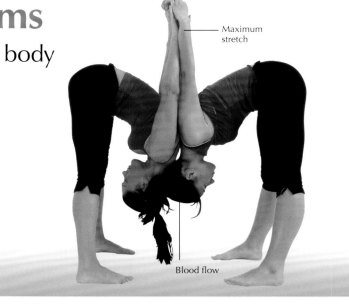

Maximum stretch

Blood flow

Benefits
- Stretches your legs, spine, and arms.
- Stretches your shoulders, triceps, and forearms.

Duration
4 to 8 breaths.

Stand face-to-face about 19 inches (50 cm) from each other, with your legs shoulder width apart, and bend forward as you bring your upper backs to touch. Stretch your arms back and intertwine your hands.

Warrior III pose
Hold, trust, and strengthen

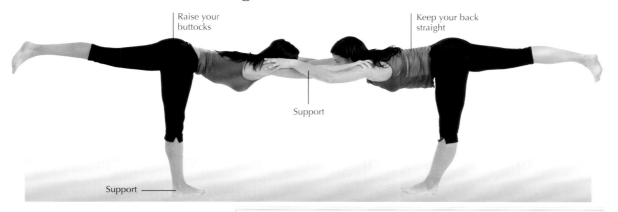

Raise your buttocks

Keep your back straight

Support

Support

Stand face-to-face about 3 feet (one meter) apart, and stand on one leg as you stretch the other leg. Stretch your arms forward and hold each other by the shoulders. Gaze into each other's eyes and sense the feelings that are aroused.

Benefits
- It strengthens the glutes, hamstrings, and the entire leg in general.
- Increases stamina and strength.

Duration
3 to 9 breaths per side. It can be repeated several times.

Tree hugging
Fusion and unity in complete privacy

Benefits
- Increases feeling of unity.
- Heat and feminine energy is shared.
- Strengthens intimacy.
- Activates erotic energy and sensuality on the skin.
- It can be said that both partners will increase their power.

Duration
Breaths: 20 to 40, at the same pace and with the same sound.

United by the first, second, third, fourth, and sixth chakras, feel energy flowing from the sexual area to the third eye. This lets many women become aware of their own bodies and erotic energy. Make contact with your toes and embrace while keeping the same breathing rate.
This asana is very powerful and can awaken the goddess within you.

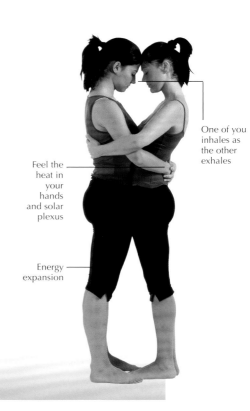

One of you inhales as the other exhales

Feel the heat in your hands and solar plexus

Energy expansion

Yogic food
"Cooking is an act of love, a gift to the beloved"

Food is one key to a successful yoga practice and renewed energy. Yoga traditionally recommends that we eat revitalizing, fresh, unprocessed foods.

Many people imagine a vegetarian kitchen as tasteless or boring; that to be a vegetarian means that you can only eat bland vegetables, but nothing could be further from the truth. Fortunately, ignorance in this regard is shrinking due to the increasing popularity of books and magazines about good nutrition.

Western foods are very heavy; our eating habits dull our senses, make our brain sluggish, and lower our energy.

Yoga is geared towards the sattvic diet that is light and full of energy, based on good "sattvic" (or "pure") food options, including all kinds of fruits, cereals, legumes, vegetables, and dairy.

Yogis regard these foods in a special way; they try to avoid "rajasic" or "stimulating" foods such as meat (including eggs), and they do not eat "tamasic" or "sedative" foods such as fried and pre-prepared meals.

In my opinion, overeating is due to anxiety caused by unfulfilled desires. This energy lies in the third chakra, and food tends to "plug" or calm our anxious energy. Remember how much you end up eating whenever you are unable to achieve a certain goal; how you wander through the kitchen whenever your energy is not geared towards something creative.

Guiding principles for eating

- Drink plenty of mineral water throughout the day—8 to 12 cups (2 to 3 liters).
- Eat only when you are hungry.
- Do not overload your stomach; leave ¼ empty with oxygen, which will speed digestion.
- Replace sausages with cereals and fried foods with fresh food.
- Do not eat if you are feeling upset. Ingesting food is a meditation.

- If you feel anxious, breathe deeply for several minutes before eating.
- Do not eat food that is too hot or too cold.
- Replace red meat with soy in any of its varieties.
- Eat fresh and dried fruit throughout the day.
- Do not mix very different foods during a meal.
- Avoid excessive fluid intake while eating.

- Brush your teeth and clean your tongue after every meal.
- Eat slowly and savor your food. Keep in mind that the digestive process begins in your mouth.
- Fast one day a week (drink water and juice, eat fruit . . .); this eliminates toxins and clears the mind.
- Prepare energizing juices.
- Gluttons and ascetics do not advance in yoga. Yoga is a luxury for intelligent people.

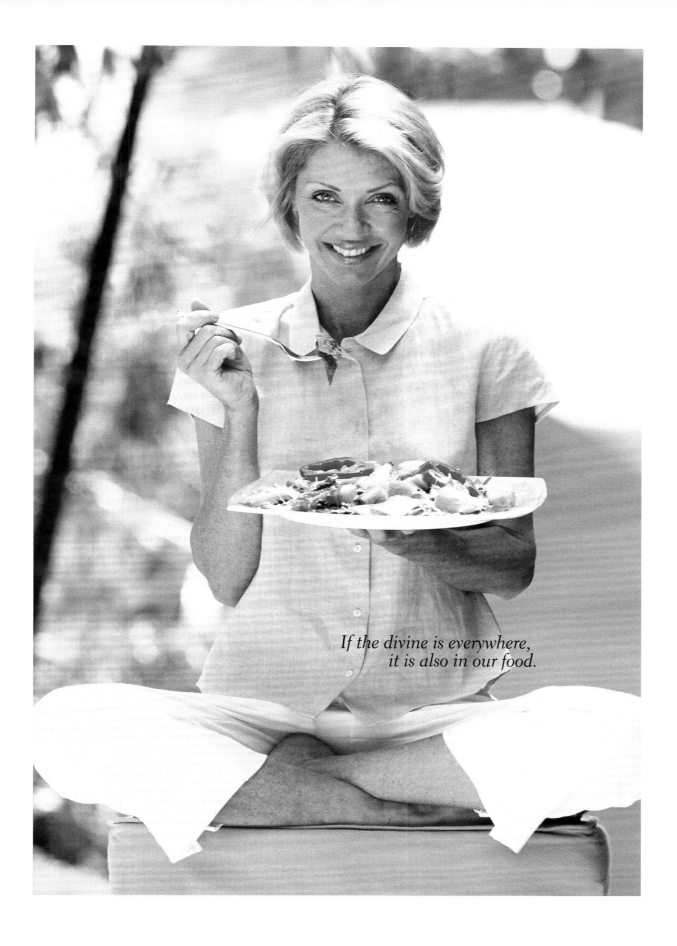

*If the divine is everywhere,
it is also in our food.*

Sattvic foods (Recommended)	Rajasic foods (excitement and stimulation)	Tamasic foods (cause laziness, clumsiness, and cloud the mind)
- Honey	- Eggs	- Red meat
- Cereals	- Refined sugar	- Fried food
- Vegetables	- Coffee	- Sausages
- Fruits	- Onion and garlic	- Frozen meals
- Juices	(eaten in small	- Canned food
- Soymilk	amounts)	- Vinegar
- Nuts	- Tobacco	
- Almonds	- Hot spices	
- Raisins	- Salt	
- Whole wheat	- Mustard	
bread	- Gherkins	
- Wheat	- Pickles	
- Brown rice		
- Oats		
- Barley		
- Corn		
- Seeds		
- Aromatic and		
medicinal plants		
- Seitan		
- Tofu		
- Tempeh		
- Celery		
- Parsley		
- Yogurt		

Knowing how to eat is an art to yoga. I am not in favor of making sacrifices and diets, or following social conventions, but I do encourage changing and substituting foods that are nothing more than empty calories for others that support and nourish us.

Do you ever ask yourself why you go to the gym? To feel healthy or to have a body that everyone can admire? Why do you sunbathe? To receive its energy or get a tan? If you live only to meet social conventions, you are damaging your body. And for yoga, your body is sacred.

Another error is poor digestion. Obviously, if you do not chew your food, if you just gobble it, there cannot be a good interaction between food and your digestive enzymes; then you do not digest properly and you feel bad.

Chewing everything you eat about sixty times is ancient yogic advice; in fact, they say you are eating God in the form of food. If you eat bread, for example, remember that it started off as a seed, which later grew, and someone's hands allowed it to come to your stomach.

If the divine is everywhere, it is also in our food.

I think that fanaticism, in whatever form, is detrimental to the health of body and mind. While there are people who obsess over religion, others fixate on food. "Guitar strings should not be too tight because they will snap, or too loose because they will not make a sound. This road requires balance," said Buddha 2,500 years ago.

It is very simple: eat when you are hungry, nourish your body with natural products, and cook your own food. When cooking, play some Pavarotti or hum along with music that inspires you and, occasionally, why not have a glass of wine? Make a feast out of every meal, celebrate every bite, feel the taste, let the appearance and aroma captivate you . . . .

Do not repress your pleasure for eating; it is the basic desire of the third chakra! If you suppress eating, sex, and love, what nice thing in life do you have left?

All that has been put on Earth is to be experienced if it challenges you to grow.

Changes that you make to your diet will help you with your yoga practice and improve the quality of your life. Personally, I never pass up a pizza and good wine*; on the contrary, you can make your own pizza using whole flour and vegetables. You won't want to have any other kind! Let yourself experience the art and pleasure of good food balanced with the wise physical and mindful exercises described in this book.

* **Editor's Note:** Traditional yoga discipline does not recommend alcohol, which is considered a "tamasic" food. Remember that yoga practice was born in India, a culture far from Mediterranean vineyards.

Yogic code for good eating

1. Chew your food thoroughly.
It is the best way to care for your digestive system. It will also help you feel satiated without overeating.

2. Eat thoughtfully.
Devote your full attention to the pleasure of eating. The digestive system reacts to the states of stress, worry, or irritation, and will not function well.

3. Taste and enjoy.
Look carefully at your plate and improve your ability to differentiate flavors. Whatever you find enjoyable will surely do you good.

4. Eat fresh fruits between meals.
Fruit offers many vitamins and fewer calories, which makes them the healthiest foods to eat between meals.

5. Stop eating prior to being full.
You need to get up from the table feeling slightly hungry. Eating moderately prolongs your life and keeps your intestinal and digestive organs healthy.

6. Eat a wide-ranging diet.
It is the best way to get all your nutrients. Take advantage of the wide variety of produce at the market and eat seasonal foods.

7. Drink when you are thirsty.
It is not true that you should not drink water with food because it dilutes the gastric juices and makes digestion difficult, although it is true that the more natural the foods, the less thirsty you will feel. You can drink red wine with meals.

8. Eat light meals.
You do not need special sauces or condiments for every meal. Make dishes that are easy to prepare.

9. Eat breakfast like an emperor, lunch like a king, and dinner like a pauper.
This would be the perfect distribution of meals in terms of quantity. At night, it is better to eat little to avoid overloading the digestive system and allow your body to take up other duties.

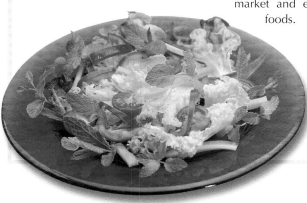

Yogic recipes
The palate can be a source of delight

"Raja" Seitan baked with vegetables

- 4 artichoke hearts
- 2 carrots
- 2 potatoes
- 2 peppers
- 1 ½ cups (150 g) of mushrooms
- Olive oil
- Soy sauce
- 10 ounces (300 g) of seitan, prepared
- 1 bunch of parsley
- Pepper
- Salt
- 1 teaspoon (5 g) of paprika
- 1 teaspoon (5 g) of curry powder

Meditate as you cook and eat consciously.

1. Preheat the oven to 350° F (180° C).
2. Julienne the vegetables.
3. In a bowl, add the olive oil, soy sauce, and vegetables; then toss to combine.
4. Season the seitan with the parsley, salt, pepper, paprika, and curry powder.
5. Bake the vegetables along with the seitan for 15-18 minutes. Once the vegetables are tender, remove them from the oven and turn the seitan over.
6. Continue to bake the seitan until it is hot throughout.

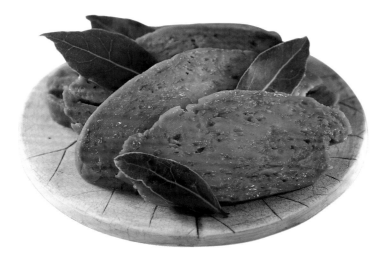

Seitan with apples and eggplants

- Chopped garlic
- Olive oil
- ¼ cup (5 g) chopped fresh cilantro
- 1 teaspoon (5 g) of ginger
- 1 cinnamon stick
- Salt
- Pepper
- 2 eggplants
- 10 ounces (300 g) of seitan
- 1 cup (¼ l) of water
- 2 apples

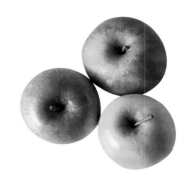

1. Cut the seitan in medium portions and marinate for 24 hours with the chopped garlic, olive oil, cilantro, ginger, cinnamon, salt, and pepper.

2. Cut the eggplant into a medium dice, season it, and let it soak in water for thirty minutes to remove bitterness. Wash and drain.

3. In a saucepan, saute the onion and the seitan for five minutes.

4. Add the water to the pan, bring to a boil, and then turn down to a steady simmer. Cover and cook for 15 minutes.

5. Peel and cut the apples into a medium dice. Add the apples and eggplant to the pan with the onions and seitan and cook for 20 minutes.

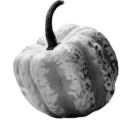

Corn and pumpkin pie

- 3 medium potatoes
- 1 lb (½ kg) pumpkin
- 2 leeks
- 2 red peppers
- 1 cup (150 g) sweet corn kernels
- Mozzarella
- Parmesan cheese
- Butter
- Olive oil

1. Preheat the oven at 350° F (180° C).
2. Peel both the potatoes and pumpkin with a knife and then cut into a large dice. Place them together into a large pot and cover with cold water. Bring to a boil and cook for 15-20 minutes or until they are very tender.
    Strain the vegetables from the water and mash together in a bowl.
3. Chop the leeks and red peppers into a medium dice.
    Add the corn, peppers, and leeks to a saute pan with olive oil and cook until softened.
4. Coat a baking dish with a thin layer of butter and add the potato and pumpkin mash in an even layer.
    Top the mash with the sautéed vegetables in a even layer and then cover with the mozzarella and Parmesan cheese.
5. Bake at 350° F (180° C) until cheese has browned nicely.

Energizing juices

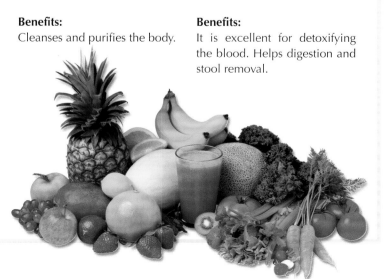

Carrot, celery, apple, and ginger juice

- 1 peeled and sliced apple
- 1 carrot, cleaned and cut into sticks
- 1 celery stalk
- ½ ginger or ¼ cup (20 g) ground ginger
- ¼ liter of mineral water

Blend all ingredients with a little water for two or three minutes until they liquefy. You can keep some in the blender to drink its pulp.

Benefits:
Carrot is rich in vitamin A and calcium. It is good for your skin, brain, digestive system, and lungs. Much like ginger, it improves circulation.

Strawberry and mint juice

- 1 ¼ cup (250 g) of strawberries
- 5 fresh mint leaves
- Pinch of cayenne pepper
- 4 teaspoons (20 g) lemon juice

Blend all the ingredients and drink instantly.

Benefits:
Cleanses and purifies the body.

Detoxifying juice

- 3 oranges
- 2 pink grapefruits
- 1 lemon
- ½ ginger root

Peel and remove the seeds of the fruit. Blend them all along with the ginger.
Drink immediately.

Benefits:
It is excellent for detoxifying the blood. Helps digestion and stool removal.

Banana mousse

- 3 bananas
- (6 oz. cups) plain yogurt
- Juice and zest of 1 lemon
- 1 teaspoon (5 g) of ginger
- 2 teaspoons (5 g) ground cinnamon
- ½ cup (125 g) of brown sugar or honey
- Unflavored gelatin or agar flakes
- 1 cup (¼ l) of water

1. Mash the bananas and mix with the yogurt.
2. Add lemon juice and zest, ginger, cinnamon, and brown sugar or honey.
3. Prepare the gelatin or agar flakes by dissolving in 1 cup (¼ l) of boiling water. Add it to the mixture and blend.
4. Pour into glasses and let cool in the refrigerator.
5. Sprinkle with cinnamon.

"Get into the habit of giving thanks for your food before eating."

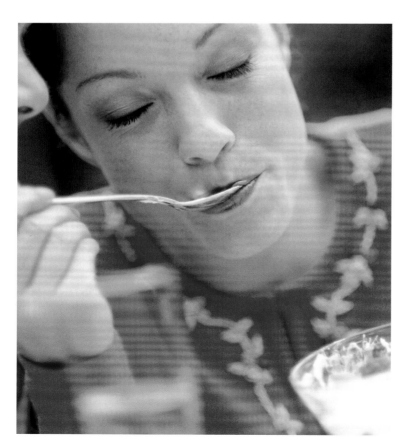

Oatmeal and pumpkin burgers

- 1 ¾ cups (250 g) soybean flour
- 1 ⅓ cups (250 g) pumpkin puree
- 2 ounces (6 cl) corn oil
- 1 teaspoon (5 g) ginger
- 2 teaspoons (5 g) paprika
- fresh parsley, chopped
- fresh oregano, chopped
- 1 ¾ cups (250 g) oat bran
- 2 teaspoons (5 g) paprika
- 2 tablespoons corn oil
- Sea salt
- Cheese

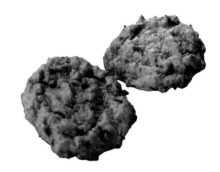

1. Combine the soybean flour with pumpkin puree and let stand for 15 minutes.
2. Meanwhile, heat a saute pan over medium-low heat and add the ginger, parsley, oregano, paprika, and salt with a tablespoon of oil.
   Heat until the spices smell fragrant.
3. To the pan, add the oat bran and the soybean and pumpkin mixture. Blend well and take off the heat. Let stand for 10 minutes.
4. Preheat the oven at 350° F (180° C).
5. Moisten your hands with water (so that they do not stick to the dough), make patties, and place them on a baking tray sprayed with non-stick spray.
6. Mix the oil with the paprika and spread it on one side of the patties.
7. Cook the patties at 350° F (180° C) and when they turn brown on one side, flip them and spread oil and paprika on the other side.
8. Once browned, lay a slice of your favorite cheese onto the patty and let melt gently. Sprinkle with oregano.

Baked tofu

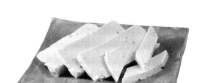

- 3 cups (500 g) tofu
- Olive oil
- Lemon juice
- Soy sauce
- Aromatic herbs (thyme, rosemary, basil, and oregano)
- Salt
- Pepper

1. Preheat the oven to 350° F (180° C).
2. Rinse the tofu, drain it, and cut it into slices ⅓ of an inch (1 cm) thick.
3. Cover a baking dish with olive oil and place the tofu in it. Sprinkle it with lemon juice, soy sauce, herbs, salt, and pepper.
4. Bake the tofu at 350 (180° C) for about thirty minutes.

Note: You can bake the tofu with a blend of aromatic herbs (thyme, rosemary, basil, and oregano), garlic, braised onion, salt, and pepper.

Recipes provided by Eliana Alonso.

Vegetable pâtés

The following pâtés are healthy and energizing, and serve as side dishes to many meals. Serve them with carrot and celery sticks, and whole wheat bread.

Avocado pâté
- 2 ripe avocados
- Juice of 1 lemon
- Olive oil
- Soy sauce
- 1 tomato, peeled and seeded
- Salt
- Pepper

Mash the avocado, and mix with tomato, lemon juice, oil, soy sauce, salt, and pepper.

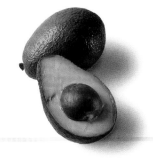

Mushroom pâté
- Olive oil
- Salt
- 3 ⅔ cups (250 g) mushrooms
- Soy sauce
- Parsley
- Aromatic herbs (thyme, rosemary, basil, and oregano)
- Toasted sesame seeds

Cut the mushrooms into thin slices, season, and fry in a pan with olive oil. Add soy sauce, parsley, and herbs, cover, and cook for about ten minutes. Finally, add the sesame seeds and grind in a food processor until a paste is achieved.

Hummus
- 1 ½ cups (250 g) cooked chickpeas
- Juice of 1 lemon
- Sesame seed oil
- Parsley

Blend chickpeas with lemon juice, sesame seed oil, and parsley. Serve immediately.

Carrot pâté
- 5 carrots
- Olive oil
- Salt
- Bay leaves
- 1 cup (125 g) ground almonds

Cut the carrots into thin slices and fry in a pan with olive oil and a little salt. Add bay leaves and a little water, and cook for ten minutes. Finally, remove the bay leaves, add the powdered almonds, and grind in a food processor until a paste is achieved.

Glossary

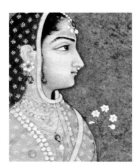

Ahamkara
Individual ego, personality mask.

Ajna
Sixth chakra, the third eye, inner ability to see clearly.

Amrita
Female ejaculation, fluid with energy properties.

Anahatta
Fourth chakra, relating to emotions and feelings.

Apana
Earth Energy.

Asana
Spiritual psychophysical posture.

Asvini Mudra
Dynamic contraction of the anus.

Atma
Individual soul.

Atman
Universal soul.

Bindu
Semen.

Brahma
Tantric God trilogy, aspect of Creation.

Brahmaranda
Opening on top of the head.

Buddha
Enlightened state of consciousness.

Chakra
Energy wheel that moves the functions of the psyche.

Chandra
Moon.

Chitta
Subconscious mind.

Dwij
Spiritual rebirth.

Hatha
Sun and moon.

Ida
Lunar duct.

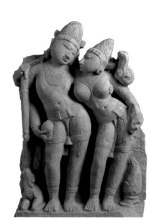

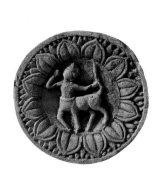

Jalandhara Bhanda
Throat lock to store energy.

Kali
Passionate, sensual, and powerful Shakti, Shiva's consort.

Kali Yuga
The Age of Kali, the present.

Kamaloka
World of desires.

Kama Sutra
Wisdom of desire, ancient Hindu treatise concerning mystical sexual secrets.

Kanda
Oval energy below the navel from which every nadis stems.

Kumbhaka
Retention of breath.

Kundalini
Sexual and mental energy stored in the first chakra.

Laksmi
Artistic aspect of women, consort of Brahma.

Lingam
Male sexual organ.

Maithuna
Sexual and mystical ritual to feel spiritual transcendence.

Mandala
Geometric diagram depicting a center. Meditation tool.

Manipura
Third chakra, solar willpower.

Mantra
Spiritual sound to still the mind.

Moksha
Spiritual liberation.

Mudra
Hand gesture to channel energy.

Mulbhand
Root lock, contracting the anal sphincter to stimulate kundalini.

Muladhara

First chakra, home of the kundalini.

Nadis

Conduits through which vital energy circulates in the body.

Nirvana

Extinction of ego, consciousness merging with the ocean of eternal life.

Ojas Shakti

Energy and spiritual power that is produced by transforming semen.

Parvati

Sweet and compassionate aspect of Shakti.

Pingala

Solar duct.

Pragna

Intuitive intelligence.

Prana

Vital energy.

Pranayamas

Techniques to absorb vital energy.

Puraka

Inhalation.

Raja

Active quality of things.

Rechaka

Exhalation.

Sahasrara

Seventh chakra, at the top of the head.

Samadhi

Dissolution of consciousness in the Whole.

Samana

One of the functions of the prana, related to excretion.

Saraswati

Consort of Vishnu.

Sattva

Bright and pure quality of things.

Shakti

Power of the feminine principle.

Shiva

God of tantric trinity, power of the male principle.

Siddhis

Extrasensory powers.

Surya

Sun.

Sushumna

Central conduit through which the kundalini rises.

Sutras

Aphorisms, teachings.

Swadisthana

Second chakra, linked to the sexual energy.

Tamas

Heavy and slow quality of things.

Udana

One of the functions of the prana, related to digestion.

Uddiyana Bandha

Lock on the abdomen, for storing energy.

Vayu

Vital air.

Vishnu

Tantric God trilogy, conservative aspect of nature.

Vishuddha

Fifth chakra, linked to creativity.

Vyana

One of the functions of prana, related to blood circulation.

Yantra

Visualization technique using power figures.

Yoga

Various energy pathways for conscious integration of the individual with the Cosmos.

Yoni

Female sexual organ.

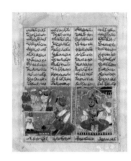

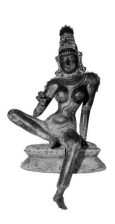